Dosage
Calculation
Workbook

ALSO FROM KAPLAN NURSING

Books

NCLEX-RN Premier with 2 Practice Tests

NCLEX-RN Strategies, Practice & Review with Practice Test

NCLEX-RN Content Review Guide

NCLEX-RN Drug Guide

NCLEX-PN Premier with 2 Practice Tests

NCLEX-PN Strategies, Practice & Review with Practice Test

NCLEX-PN Content Review Guide

First Year Nurse

Adult CCRN Strategies, Practice & Review with 2 Practice Tests

Online

Kaplan NCLEX-RN Qbank

Kaplan NCLEX-PN Qbank

Dosage Calculation Workbook

MATH REVIEW AND PRACTICE FOR NURSES

Edited by

Bart Brinkmann, DNP, ARNP, FNP-C

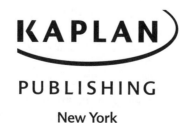

KAPLAN

PUBLISHING

New York

© 2016 by Kaplan, Inc.

Published by Kaplan Publishing, a division of Kaplan, Inc.
750 Third Avenue
New York, NY 10017

10 9 8 7 6 5 4 3 2 1

ISBN-13: 978-1-5062-0802-2

Kaplan Publishing books are available at special quantity discounts to use for sales promotions, employee premiums, or educational purposes. For more information or to purchase books, please call the Simon & Schuster special sales department at 866-506-1949.

Contents

Contributors

Bart Brinkmann, DNP, ARNP, FNP-C, is a family nurse practitioner and experienced cardiac ICU RN. While pursuing his Doctor of Nursing Practice degree through Washington State University, he taught medical/surgical nursing and dosage calculation to undergraduate nursing students. He currently works for a community-owned cardiology practice and provides both inpatient and outpatient cardiac care.

Kaplan thanks the following experts for their contributions to this book, previously entitled *Math for Nurses*:

Mary E. Stassi
Margaret A. Tiemann

Introduction

Electronic Health Record (EHR) software, used in most hospitals and clinics, automatically calculates dosages and tells the nurse how many pills or milliliters to administer to their patients. An EHR saves nurses a great deal of time and significantly improves patient safety, but it doesn't make dosage calculation any less important. Computer systems go down, medication orders can change at a moment's notice, and new medications must often be given before an order can be entered and verified in an EHR. Regardless of how much technology changes, dosage calculation will always be a core nursing skill.

Kaplan's *Dosage Calculation Workbook* is a comprehensive guide for aspiring and experienced nurses alike. Whether learning to calculate drug dosages for the first time, reviewing for certification, or referencing for a specific calculation, readers will appreciate the clear, concise organization of this easy-to-use text. Information is organized in a logical manner that progresses from basic mathematical principles to complex dosage calculation.

This book includes:

- Practice problems
- Easy-to-follow examples
- Step-by-step explanations
- Math tips from experienced nurse educators
- Chapter quizzes designed to test your mastery of math topics
- Answer keys conveniently located at the end of each chapter

How to Use This Book

Kaplan's *Dosage Calculation Workbook* starts with a 30-question diagnostic test designed to assess the basic math skills required for dosage calculation. The diagnostic correlation chart at the end of the test will help you identify your strengths and weaknesses. After completing this short test, you may choose to spend time reviewing the foundational skills in Part 1. (Those who score a 90% or better on the diagnostic test may be comfortable proceeding straight to Part 2.) Part 1 is divided into six chapters and provides an in-depth review of the core skills required for dosage calculation. Once you feel comfortable with these foundational math skills, you will be ready to move on to Part 2, where you will learn conversions and dosage calculation.

Part 1: Foundational Skills

Part 1 offers a comprehensive, step-by-step guide to solving equations with pen and paper. While calculators have their place in the clinical setting, being able to solve these foundational arithmetic problems by hand will increase your confidence, and often it's faster and more accurate than using a calculator or computer.

Chapter 1 reviews the four math basics: addition, subtraction, multiplication, and division.

Chapter 2 explains fractions. In this chapter, you will practice adding, subtracting, multiplying, and dividing fractions. Reducing fractions and dealing with mixed numbers will also be covered.

Chapter 3 is a review of the decimal system, which is the foundation of the metric system. In this chapter you will learn how to add, subtract, multiply, and divide decimals. This chapter also covers converting fractions to decimals and decimals to fractions.

Chapter 4 covers percentages and how to convert between fractions, decimals, and percentages.

Chapter 5 explains ratios and proportions, which are commonly used to calculate medication dosages.

Chapter 6 is a review of rates and how they are used to calculate flow, which is important for dealing with IV medications.

Part 2: Applications

Part 2 uses the foundations reviewed in Part 1 to calculate dosages based on medication orders. After covering the various systems of measurement used for dosing medications, you will learn three methods for calculating doses for oral and parenteral medications.

Chapter 7 discusses the three systems of measurement used in medicine: metric, apothecary, and household. Accurately converting between these three systems will help to ensure safe, error-free administration of medications.

Chapter 8 introduces the three methods used for dosage calculation: ratio-proportion, formula, and dimensional analysis. Since each method will yield the same answer, you can choose the method you prefer to calculate all your dosage problems—and you are sure to develop a preference as you progress. Note that using two different methods on each problem is a reliable method for checking your answers.

Chapter 9 focuses on calculating dosages for oral administration of pills and liquids.

Chapter 10 introduces parenteral medication administration. This chapter focuses on injections.

Chapter 11 covers dosage calculation for the various modes of intravenous drug administration.

Chapter 12 discusses age-specific considerations for dosing medications based on body weight and body surface area. These considerations are particularly important in pediatric and geriatric populations.

> **Math Tip:** Remember, before you solve your equation, take a moment to confirm that all information in your problem is correct and is in the proper location. Get in the habit of reviewing your problem just before you solve, and you will significantly reduce your margin of error.

1 Foundation Skills

Diagnostic Test

The 30-question diagnostic test is designed to help you identify the areas you need to review. Find a comfortable and quiet place with good lighting to take the test. Select a time when you will not be interrupted, and allow at least 30 minutes to take the test. Solve each of the problems *without* using a calculator. If you don't know an answer, skip it, go on with the rest of the test, and come back to it later. Keep a positive attitude throughout the whole test and try to stay relaxed; if you start to feel nervous, take a few deep breaths to relax.

When you have finished, compare your answers with the answer key. The correlation chart will indicate which area(s) you should review before moving on to Part 2 of the book. The practice problems in each chapter provide step-by-step explanations and will help you to work through the chapter. Complete the chapter quizzes and check your answers. Go back and rework any problems that you got wrong before moving on. Even if you do well on the diagnostic test, reviewing Chapters 1–6 will help get your brain functioning in "math mode" and sharpen your basic arithmetic skills as you prepare to review the applications chapters in Part 2.

If you score 90 percent or better on the diagnostic test, you may decide to skip Part 1 and begin with Chapter 7: Systems of Measurement. However, if at any time you feel the need to review anything from Part 1, go back to the appropriate chapter and look over the example problems again.

DIRECTIONS

Each question below is followed by four possible answers. Select the best answer for each question and circle the letter. Try to complete the entire diagnostic test in 30 minutes.

1. $1,534 + 201 + 888 + 45 =$

   (A) 2,668   (C) 2,768

   (B) 2,566   (D) 2,868

2. $4,578 - 987 =$

   (A) 2,591   (C) 3,591

   (B) 3,011   (D) 3,781

3. $456 \times 27 =$

   (A) 9,422   (C) 11,468

   (B) 10,329   (D) 12,312

4. $11,487 \div 547 =$

   (A) 12   (C) 27

   (B) 21   (D) 31

5. $15,604 \div 47 =$

   (A) 332   (C) 404

   (B) 392   (D) 522

6. $\dfrac{3}{18} \times \dfrac{6}{9} =$

    (A) $\dfrac{9}{162}$ (C) $\dfrac{1}{2}$

    (B) $\dfrac{1}{9}$ (D) $\dfrac{18}{27}$

7. $\dfrac{3}{8} + \dfrac{16}{24} =$

    (A) $\dfrac{19}{32}$ (C) 2

    (B) $1\dfrac{1}{24}$ (D) $2\dfrac{2}{3}$

8. $\dfrac{105}{42}$ reduced to the simplest form is

    (A) $1\dfrac{1}{6}$ (C) $2\dfrac{1}{2}$

    (B) $1\dfrac{1}{2}$ (D) $2\dfrac{1}{3}$

9. $\dfrac{1}{75} \div \dfrac{1}{150} =$

    (A) $\dfrac{1}{4}$ (C) $1\dfrac{1}{2}$

    (B) $\dfrac{1}{2}$ (D) 2

10. $\dfrac{3}{5} =$

    (A) 0.3   (C) 0.6

    (B) 0.35   (D) 3.5

11. $6.5 \times 0.2 =$

    (A) 1.3   (C) 12.5

    (B) 6.1   (D) 13

12. $0.0421 =$

    (A) $\dfrac{421}{10}$ (C) $\dfrac{421}{1,000}$

    (B) $\dfrac{421}{100}$ (D) $\dfrac{421}{10,000}$

13. $3.42 \div 34.2 =$

    (A) 0.1   (C) 1

    (B) 0.342   (D) 34.2

14. $6 + 2.8 + 1.7 =$

    (A) 1.04   (C) 10.5

    (B) 10.4   (D) 105

15. $165.55 - 83.97 =$

    (A) 61.88   (C) 81.58

    (B) 71.48   (D) 91.68

16. Convert $\frac{2}{5}$ to a percentage.

    (A) 20%   (C) 60%

    (B) 40%   (D) 80%

17. 0.375 = _____%

    (A) 0.375   (C) 37.5

    (B) 3.75   (D) 375

18. What is 60% of 300?

    (A) 80   (C) 180

    (B) 160   (D) 260

19. 10 is what percentage of 400?

    (A) 0.025%   (C) 2.5%

    (B) 0.25%   (D) 25%

20. What number is 14% of 88?

    (A) 0.76   (C) 12.32

    (B) 7.98   (D) 22.96

21. If $\frac{2}{3} = \frac{x}{9}$, then $x =$

    (A) 1   (C) 4
    (B) 2   (D) 6

22. If $\frac{4\,mg}{0.8\,mL} = \frac{x\,mg}{2\,mL}$, then $x =$

    (A) 0.1   (C) 10
    (B) 0.4   (D) 16

23. A patient is to receive 35 mg of a certain medication at 70 mg per mL of solution. How much of the solution should be given?

    (A) 0.35 mL   (C) 2 mL
    (B) 0.5 mL   (D) 5 mL

24. $4 : 7 :: 12 : x$; therefore, $x =$

    (A) 8   (C) 21
    (B) 16   (D) 28

25. The proportion $1 : 10 :: 3 : 30$ can be restated in fraction form as which of the following?

    (A) $\frac{1}{10} = \frac{30}{3}$ (C) $\frac{3}{10} = \frac{1}{30}$
    (B) $\frac{10}{1} = \frac{3}{30}$ (D) $\frac{1}{10} = \frac{3}{30}$

26. The physician orders 1,000 mL of IV fluids to infuse over 8 hours. How many mL per hour must infuse?

    (A) 100 mL　　　　(C) 150 mL
    (B) 125 mL　　　　(D) 175 mL

27. The physician orders 1,000 mL of IV fluids to infuse over 8 hours. The drop factor for the IV tubing is 15 gtts/mL. How many gtts/min should infuse?

    (A) 10　　　　(C) 30
    (B) 20　　　　(D) 40

28. A patient is scheduled to receive 500 mL of TPN solution over the next 10 hours. The IV set delivers 60 drops per mL. How many drops should the patient receive per minute?

    (A) 12　　　　(C) 50
    (B) 42　　　　(D) 125

29. You need to infuse a total of 3,000 mL of IV fluids. If the flow rate is set at 125 mL/hr, how long will it take to infuse the total amount?

    (A) 15 hours　　　　(C) 24 hours
    (B) 20 hours　　　　(D) 30 hours

30. The patient is to receive 250 mL of packed red blood cells over three hours using an electronic infusion pump. What rate should the pump should be programmed at?

    (A) 83.33 mL/hr　　　　(C) 112.75 mL/hr
    (B) 97.5 mL/hr　　　　(D) 125 mL/hr

DIAGNOSTIC TEST ANSWER KEY

1.	A	16.	B
2.	C	17.	C
3.	D	18.	C
4.	B	19.	C
5.	A	20.	C
6.	B	21.	D
7.	B	22.	C
8.	C	23.	B
9.	D	24.	C
10.	C	25.	D
11.	A	26.	B
12.	D	27.	C
13.	A	28.	C
14.	C	29.	C
15.	C	30.	A

Correct your test using this key. Then refer to the correlation chart that follows to determine whether you need to complete all of Part 1: Foundation Skills, just particular chapters, or no review at all. Answer explanations are provided at the end of this chapter.

Part 1 is designed to provide a refresher course on the essential math concepts used for dosage calculations. Part 2: Applications will give you an opportunity to work on problems with real-life applications.

DIAGNOSTIC TEST CORRELATION CHART

Directions: Calculate the number of questions you answered correctly in each section. This will help you to determine where you need to focus your review.

Section	Number of Questions Answered Correctly
Basic Arithmetic Questions 1–5	0–1: You need some review in solving basic arithmetic problems. You should review Chapter 1 before moving on.
	2–3: You seem to have an understanding of the basics. Go back and double-check your answers, paying close attention to multiplication and division questions.
	4–5: Terrific! You have a good understanding of the foundations of all math problems.

(continued)

Section	Number of Questions Answered Correctly
Fractions Questions 6–10	0–1: You need some review in working with fractions. Start at the beginning of Chapter 2 and follow each of the example problems before trying to solve the practice questions.
	2–3: You've got a pretty good grasp of fractions, but a review of Chapter 2 would help strengthen your skills in this area.
	4–5: Very good! Fractions don't intimidate you. Feel free to move on to decimals.
Decimals Questions 11–15	0–1: You need to work on decimals. Chapter 3 is an excellent review and will get you moving in the right direction.
	2–3: OK, but you still need some work. Review Chapter 3 to reinforce your abilities.
	4–5: Nice job! You have a good understanding of decimals. This will help you as you work on more difficult calculations.
Percentages Questions 16–20	0–1: Percentages can be tough. Complete the practice problems and end-of-chapter quiz for Chapter 4.
	2–3: You are about halfway (or 50 percent) there! Spend some time reviewing Chapter 4 before you move on.
	4–5: Very good! You understand the concept of percentages and can work some challenging problems.
Ratios Questions 21–25	0–1: Chapter 5 is a "must." Take time to review the practice problems to understand better how to set up the ratios. Make sure that your basic arithmetic is correct as well.
	2–3: You are moving in the right direction but still need to review. Chapter 5 should give you what you need to gain confidence with ratios and proportions.
	4–5: Now you've got it! These were some tough questions. Give yourself a pat on the back if you got all five questions correct.
Rates Questions 26–30	0–1: Rates can be difficult to calculate, but Chapter 6 is a terrific review. Start at the beginning and work each practice problem.
	2–3: Not too bad, but you could use a little bit of review. Chapter 6 should give you what you need.
	4–5: Great! Determining rates is one of the hardest calculations for most nurses. Keep up the good work.

DIAGNOSTIC TEST ANSWERS AND EXPLANATIONS

1. A

Begin by rewriting the problem with the numbers in a column. Remember to line up, or justify, the numbers to the right. Add each column starting with the ones, then the tens, and so on. Remember to carry over to the next column as needed.

$$
\begin{array}{r}
1,534 \\
201 \\
888 \\
+\quad 45 \\
\hline
2,668
\end{array}
$$

2. C

When subtracting numbers, remember to rewrite the problem using a column. Justify the columns to the right so that the ones, tens, hundreds, and thousands places line up. Begin by subtracting the ones, then the tens, etc. Borrow from the next column to the left when the bottom number in the problem is larger than the top number.

$$
\begin{array}{r}
4,578 \\
-\quad 987 \\
\hline
3,591
\end{array}
$$

3. D

Begin by rewriting the problem in a column. Multiply the first digit (in the ones column) of the bottom number by the entire top number. Write the product under the line. Remember to carry numbers over if needed. Next, multiply the second number (tens column) by the entire top number. Write the product under the line, moving one place to the left. Add the products together for the correct answer.

$$
\begin{array}{r}
456 \\
\times\quad 27 \\
\hline
3,192 \\
9\ 12\quad \\
\hline
12,312
\end{array}
$$

4. B

Convert the problem to long division format by placing the divisor (the number you are dividing by) before the division bracket and the dividend (the number you are dividing into) under it. Solve the problem by dividing the number inside of the bracket, the dividend, by the number outside of the bracket, the divisor. Subtract each number as you solve the problem. The answer, or quotient, is written on top of the bracket.

$$
\begin{array}{r}
21 \\
547\overline{)11,487} \\
-1,094 \\
\hline
547 \\
-\ 547 \\
\hline
0
\end{array}
$$

5. A

Convert the problem to long division format by placing the divisor (the number you are dividing by) before the division bracket and the dividend (the number you are dividing into) under it. Solve the problem by dividing the number inside of the bracket, the dividend, by the number outside of the bracket, the divisor. Subtract each number as you solve the problem. The answer (quotient) is written on top of the bracket.

$$
\begin{array}{r}
332 \\
47\overline{)15,604} \\
-141 \\
\hline
150 \\
-\ 141 \\
\hline
94 \\
-\ 94 \\
\hline
0
\end{array}
$$

6. B

To multiply fractions, simply multiply the numerators (top numbers) and then multiply the denominators (bottom numbers) to find the product.

$$3 \times 6 = 18$$
$$18 \times 9 = 162$$

Reduce the answer to its lowest terms or simplest form.

$$\frac{18}{162} = \frac{1}{9}$$

7. B

After finding the common denominator (in this problem, 24), add the numerators (top numbers). Write the sum over the denominator.

$$\frac{3}{8} = \frac{9}{24}$$

$$\frac{9}{24} + \frac{16}{24} = \frac{25}{24}$$

Reduce the answer.

$$\frac{25}{24} = 1\frac{1}{24}$$

8. C

Determine the largest number by which both the numerator (top number) and denominator (bottom number) can be divided equally; in this problem, that number is 21. Divide both the numerator and denominator by 21.

$$105 \div 21 = 5$$
$$42 \div 21 = 2$$

Reduce the answer.

$$\frac{5}{2} = 2\frac{1}{2}$$

9. D

Set up the problem. When dividing fractions, you must first invert the second fraction (switch the top and bottom numbers) and then multiply the fractions.

Reduce the answer to its lowest terms, converting it from an improper fraction (i.e., the numerator is greater than the denominator) to a whole number.

$$\frac{1}{75} \div \frac{1}{150} = \frac{1}{75} \times \frac{150}{1} = \frac{150}{75} = 2$$

10. C

Divide the numerator (top number) by the denominator (bottom number).

$$3 \div 5 = .6$$

Add a zero to the left of the decimal point, so .6 becomes 0.6 and is clearer to read.

11. A

Write the problem with the greater number of digits (multiplicand) above the number with the smaller number of digits (multiplier). You may drop the zero in the bottom number since it is to the left of the decimal point. Multiply the digit farthest to the right of the multiplier by each of the digits of the multiplicand. Carry numbers as necessary to the next place to the left. Count the number of decimal places in both the multiplicand and the multiplier. In this problem, there are two. Starting from the right in the answer, count two to the left and insert the decimal point. This is the final answer, or product.

$$\begin{array}{r} 6.5 \\ \times\ 0.2 \\ \hline 1.30 \end{array}$$

12. D

Remove the decimal point and place the decimal number over whatever number is denoted by the place of the last digit. This fraction cannot be reduced.

$$\frac{421}{10,000}$$

13. A

Move the decimal point of the divisor to the end of the number, making it a whole number. Move the decimal point in the dividend the same number of spaces as the decimal point was moved in the divisor. Place a decimal point in the quotient line directly above the decimal point in the dividend line. Divide the numbers, adding zeros to the end of the dividend as needed. The answer, or quotient, is 0.1.

$$3.42 \div 34.2 \text{ becomes } 342\overline{)34.2} \\ \underline{-34.2} \\ 0 \quad (0.1)$$

14. C

Carefully write all decimal numbers in a column, aligning the numbers and decimal points directly beneath each other and in a straight line. To make things easier, trailing zeros may be used to help keep the columns justified. In this problem, a trailing zero was added to 6 to make it 6.0. Bring the decimal point down below the sum or answer line. Add the numbers in each column.

$$\begin{array}{r} 6.0 \\ 2.8 \\ +\ 1.7 \\ \hline 10.5 \end{array}$$

15. C

Carefully write the decimal numbers in columns, aligning the numbers and decimal points directly beneath each other and in a straight line. Bring the decimal point down to below the answer line. Subtract the numbers in each column, borrowing from the next column to the left if necessary.

$$\begin{array}{r} 165.55 \\ -\ 83.97 \\ \hline 81.58 \end{array}$$

16. B

To convert a fraction to a percent, multiply the fraction by 100.

$$\frac{2 \times 100}{5 \times 1} = \frac{200}{5}$$

Reduce to $\frac{40}{1} = 40$ and add the percent symbol (%). The correct answer is 40%.

17. C

To change a decimal to a percent, multiply the decimal by 100. This requires you to move the decimal point two places to the right. Add percent symbol (%).

$$0.375 \times 100 = 37.5$$

37.5% is the correct answer.

18. C

This problem is best set up as a ratio-proportion that requires you to solve for x.

Cross multiply to get the product of the means and the extremes. Divide both sides of the proportion by the number in front of the x, 100. (The number in front of x is called the *coefficient*.)

$$\frac{60}{100} \diagdown \frac{x}{300}$$

$60 \times 300 = 18{,}000$, and $100 \times x = 100x$. $18{,}000 \div 100 = 180$, and $100x \div 100 = x$, so $180 = x$.

This means that 180 is 60% of 300.

19. C

This problem is best set up as a ratio-proportion that requires you to solve for *x*.

Cross multiply to get the product of the means and the extremes. Divide both sides of the proportion by the number in front of the *x*, 400. Don't forget to turn the fraction into a percentage at the end, or your answer will be incorrect!

$$\frac{10}{400} \diagup\!\!\!\!\diagup \frac{x}{100}$$

$10 \times 100 = 1{,}000$, and $400 \times x = 400x$.
$1{,}000 \div 400 = 2.5$, and $400x \div 400 = x$, so $2.5 = x$.

Now calculate the percentage: $\frac{2.5}{100}$ becomes 0.025, or 2.5%.

20. C

This problem is best set up as a ratio-proportion that requires you to solve for *x*.

Cross multiply to get the product of the means and the extremes. Divide both sides of the proportion by the number in front of the *x*, 100.

$$\frac{14}{100} \diagup\!\!\!\!\diagup \frac{x}{88}$$

$14 \times 88 = 1{,}232$, and $100 \times x = 100x$.
$1{,}232 \div 100 = 12.32$, and $100x \div 100 = x$, so $12.32 = x$.

This means that 12.32 is 14% of 88.

21. D

Cross multiply to get the product of the means and the extremes. Divide both sides of the proportion by the number in front of the *x*, 3.

$$\frac{2}{3} \diagup\!\!\!\!\diagup \frac{x}{9}$$

$2 \times 9 = 18$, and, $3 \times x = 3x$.
$18 \div 3 = 6$, and $3x \div 3 = x$, so $6 = x$.

22. C

Cross multiply to get the product of the means and the extremes. Divide both sides of the proportion by the number in front of the *x*, 0.8. Make sure that *mg* appears above the line on both sides and *mL* appears below the line to get an accurate answer. After the problem is set up, you may disregard the *mg* and *mL* references while solving the math equation.

$$\frac{4\ \text{mg}}{0.8\ \text{mL}} \diagup\!\!\!\!\diagup \frac{x\ \text{mg}}{2\ \text{mL}}$$

$4 \times 2 = 8$, and $0.8 \times x = 0.8x$.
$8 \div 0.8 = 10$, and $0.8x \div 0.8 = x$, so $10 = x$.

23. B

You must first determine the appropriate method of setting up the problem. This means determining what you already know and what you need to find out. In this problem, you know that there is 70 mg of drug per 1 mL of solution. You want to give 35 mg of the drug and need to know how many mL of solution to give.

Cross multiply to get the product of the means and the extremes. Divide both sides of the proportion by the number in front of the *x*, 70. Make sure that *mg* appears above the line on both sides and *mL* below the line to get an accurate answer. After the problem is set up, you may disregard the *mg* and *mL* references while solving the math equation.

$$\frac{70\ \text{mg}}{1\ \text{mL}} \diagup\!\!\!\!\diagup \frac{35\ \text{mg}}{x\ \text{mL}}$$

$70 \times x = 70x$, and $1 \times 35 = 35$.
$70x \div 70 = x$, and $35 \div 70 = 0.5$, so $x = 0.5$.

You would give 0.5 mL of the solution.

24. C

Multiply the means and the extremes.

$7 \times 12 = 84$ (means)

$4 \times x = 4x$ (extremes)

Therefore:

$84 = 4x$

Divide both sides of the equation by the number in front of the x: 4.

$4x \div 4 = x$

$84 \div 4 = 21$

Therefore:

$x = 21$

25. D

When converting between ratios and fractions, no calculations are necessary. Simply change the way the numbers are presented. Replace the double colon (::) with an equal sign (=).

$1 : 10 = \dfrac{1}{10}$, and $3 : 30 = \dfrac{3}{30}$

So $1 : 10 :: 3 : 30$ is the same as $\dfrac{1}{10} = \dfrac{3}{30}$.

26. B

Determine what you already know and what you need to find out. In this problem, you know that you will infuse 1,000 mL of fluid over eight hours. You need to know how many mL of fluid will be given in one hour.

Cross multiply to get the product of the means and the extremes. Divide both sides of proportion by the number in front of the x, 8. Make sure that *mL* appears above the line on both sides and *hours* below the line to get an accurate answer. After the problem is set up, you may disregard the *hour* and *mL* references while solving the math equation.

$$\frac{1{,}000 \text{ mL}}{8 \text{ hours}} \diagup\!\!\!\!\diagdown \frac{x \text{ mL}}{1 \text{ hour}}$$

$1{,}000 \times 1 = 1{,}000$, and $8 \times x = 8x$.

$1{,}000 \div 8 = 125$, and $8x \div 8 = x$, so $125 = x$.

You would infuse 125 mL of fluid per hour.

27. C

This problem requires you to determine two different things. How many mL per minute should infuse must be determined before you can calculate the number of drops per minute. Question 26 shows how to determine the number of mL per hour that would infuse if you are infusing 1,000 mL in eight hours.

Since you already know that you must give 125 mL in one hour (60 minutes), it is easy to go one step farther and determine how many mL to give in one minute by solving for x. Cross multiply to get the product of the means and the extremes. Divide both sides of the proportion by the number in front of the x, 60. Make sure that *mL* appears above the line on both sides and *minutes* below the line to get an accurate answer. After the problem is set up, you may disregard the *minute* and *mL* references while solving the math equation.

$$\frac{125 \text{ mL}}{60 \text{ minutes}} \diagup\!\!\!\!\diagdown \frac{x \text{ mL}}{1 \text{ minute}}$$

$125 \times 1 = 125$, and $60 \times x = 60x$.

$125 \div 60 = 2.083$, and $60x \div 60 = x$,

so $2.083 = x$.

This answer would be rounded to 2.

The second part of the problem requires you to solve for x again. You know that there are 15 drops in 1 mL, and you need to know how many drops are in 2 mL. You can do this part easily.

$$\frac{15 \text{ drops}}{1 \text{ mL}} \diagup\!\!\!\!\diagdown \frac{x \text{ drops}}{2 \text{ mL}}$$

Cross multiply to get $30 = x$.

Therefore, 30 gtts/min should infuse.

28. C

This problem requires you to determine two different things. How many mL per minute should infuse must be determined before you can calculate the number of drops per minute. You know that you are going to give 500 mL of TPN solution over 10 hours. Since there are 60 minutes in an hour, this is the same as 500 mL in 600 minutes. You can now set up the problem to determine how many drops the patient will receive per minute.

$$\frac{500 \text{ mL}}{600 \text{ min}} \diagup\!\!\!\!\diagdown \frac{x \text{ mL}}{1 \text{ min}}$$

Cross multiply.

$500 \times 1 = 500$, and $600 \times x = 600x$.

Divide both sides by the number in front of the x, 600.

$500 \div 600 = 0.83$, and
$600x \div 600 = x$, so $0.83 = x$.

You now know that the patient should receive 0.83 mL per minute. You can complete the next step since you also know that the IV set delivers 60 drops per mL.

$$\frac{60 \text{ drops}}{1 \text{ mL}} \diagup\!\!\!\!\diagdown \frac{x \text{ drops}}{0.83 \text{ mL}}$$

Cross multiply, ignoring the mL and drops at this time.

$60 \times 0.83 = 49.8$, and $1 \times x = 1x$.

Divide both sides by the number in front of the x, 1.

$x = 49.8$

Since it is not possible to give part of a drop, this would be rounded up to 50. The patient will receive 50 drops/minute.

29. C

Determine what you already know and what you need to find out. In this problem, you know that you will infuse 125 mL of fluid every hour. You need to know how long it will take to infuse 3,000 mL of fluid.

Cross multiply to get the product of the means and the extremes. Divide both sides of the proportion by the number in front of the x, 125. Make sure that *mL* appears above the line on both sides and *hours* below the line to get an accurate answer. After the problem is set up, you may disregard the *hour* and *mL* references while solving the math equation.

$$\frac{125 \text{ mL}}{1 \text{ hour}} \diagup\!\!\!\!\diagdown \frac{3,000 \text{ mL}}{x \text{ hours}}$$

$125 \times x = 125x$, and $1 \times 3,000 = 3,000$.
$125x \div 125 = x$, and $3,000 \div 125 = 24$,
so $x = 24$.

It will take 24 hours to infuse the 3,000 mL of fluid.

30. A

Determine what you already know and what you need to find out. In this problem, you know that you will infuse 250 mL of packed red blood cells over three hours. You need to know how many mL per hour will infuse to correctly set the pump.

Cross multiply to get the product of the means and the extremes. Divide both sides of the proportion by the number in front of the x, 3. Make sure that *mL* appears above the line on both sides and *hours* below the line to get an accurate answer. After the problem is set up, you may disregard the *hour* and *mL* references while solving the math equation.

$$\frac{250 \text{ mL}}{3 \text{ hours}} = \frac{x \text{ mL}}{1 \text{ hour}}$$

$250 \times 1 = 250$, and $3 \times x = 3x$.
$250 \div 3 = 83.33$, and $3x \div 3 = x$,
so $83.33 = x$.

The pump should be set at 83.33 mL/hr if the setting will permit it. If you must round, the rate would be rounded to 83 mL/hr.

CHAPTER 1

Basic Arithmetic

Addition, subtraction, multiplication, and division form the foundation for nearly every clinical decision you'll make as a nurse. Whether you're balancing intake and output, trending vital signs, or titrating a pediatric dopamine infusion, there's always some form of basic arithmetic involved. As mundane as it may sound, mastering these core concepts is essential for accurately processing the information you will collect, record, and act on throughout your day. Before diving into the more advanced concepts and formulas you'll be using as a nurse, take this opportunity to brush up on the basic arithmetic skills that you will use over the course of this book.

Addition

Addition is simply the process of adding something to something else. When adding two or more numbers together, the result is referred to as the *sum*.

For example, 4 + 2 = 6; therefore, 6 is the sum of the addition of 4 and 2.

Working with numbers in columns or rows makes solving the problem easier.

Example: 2,235 + 75 + 123 = 2,433

```
   2,235
      75
 +  123
   2,433
```

Each column has a place value. Moving from the right to the left, the first place is the "ones" column, the second is the "tens," the third is the "hundreds," the fourth is the "thousands," and so on.

> **Math Tip:** When adding whole numbers, it is important to justify the columns to the right so that the ones, tens, hundreds, and thousands places, or columns, line up correctly.

```
  2,235
     75
+   123
  2,433
```

Notice that the bold numbers are justified, or lined up in a column. Failure to justify the numbers can result in an incorrect answer or sum.

Now that the problem is set up correctly, following the steps below to review how to obtain the correct answer.

First, add the numbers in the ones column: $5 + 5 + 3 = 13$. Since 13 is more than 9, the maximum number that can be listed in this column, the 3 is placed under the line, and the 1 is carried over into the tens column.

```
     1
  2,235
     75
+   123
      3
```

Next, add the tens column, remembering to add in the 1 carried over from the previous column ($3 + 7 + 2 + 1 = 13$). The 3 is again placed below the line, and the 1 is carried over to the next column to the left.

```
    1 1
  2,235
     75
+   123
     33
```

Continue by adding the numbers in the hundreds column, remembering to add in the number carried over ($2 + 1 + 1 = 4$).

```
    1 1
  2,235
     75
+   123
    433
```

Notice that the numbers under the line (those in the sum) are also aligned to justify to the right so that they appear in the correct column.

```
    1 1
  2,235
     75
+   123
  2,433
```

Practice 1

1. 147 + 98 =

2. 498 + 561 =

3. 326 + 75 + 9 =

4. 1,362 + 732 + 89 + 15 =

5. 2,358 + 863 + 85 + 4 =

Subtraction

Subtraction is the opposite, or inverse, of addition. When subtracting, one number is taken away from another. The result of subtraction is referred to as the *difference*.

For example, 7 – 4 = 3; therefore, 3 is the difference between 7 and 4, and 3 + 4 = 7.

Working with numbers in columns makes solving subtraction problems easier. As with addition, justify the columns to the right so that the ones, tens, hundreds, and thousands places line up correctly.

Example: 427 – 81 = ?

```
   427
 –  81
 ─────
```

Now that the problem is set up correctly, follow the steps below to obtain the correct answer. First, subtract the bottom number in the ones column from the top number in that column (7 – 1 = 6). The 6 is placed below the line in the correct column.

```
   427
 –  81
 ─────
     6
```

Next, subtract the tens column (2 – 8 = ?). Since 8 is larger than 2, it is not possible to complete this calculation unless we borrow from the next column to the left. Cross out the 4 and write 3 to borrow 10, and add it to our 2 to get 12 (12 – 8 = 4). The 4 is placed under the line in the tens column.

```
   3 12
  4̶2̶7
-  81
  ----
   46
```

Lastly subtract the hundreds column. Since there is no number to subtract in the hundreds column, the number simply moves down. Remember that 1 was borrowed from the 4, so it became a 3 in the last step.

```
   3 12
  4̶2̶7
-  81
  ----
  346
```

Practice 2

1. 54 – 17 =

2. 296 – 43 =

3. 720 – 316 =

4. 3,859 – 532 =

5. 8,365 – 3,976 =

Multiplication

Multiplication is nothing more than repeated addition. When multiplying two numbers together, you pick one number and choose how many times to repeat it. The number to be repeated, or multiplied, is referred to as the *multiplicand*. The other number in the equation, the *multiplier*, determines how many times the multiplicand is repeated. The result when two numbers are multiplied together is referred to as the *product*.

When you look at an equation like $3 \times 5 = 15$, it can difficult to understand the rationale for referring to the 3 as the multiplicand and the 5 as the multiplier, because in this case either number can be referred to as either the multiplicand or the multiplier. You can add the number 3 together 5 times, or you can add the number 5 together 3 times, and either way you end up with the same product of 15.

$$3 + 3 + 3 + 3 + 3 = 15 \qquad 5 + 5 + 5 = 15$$

When you start dealing with repeating actions or medication doses, however, these nuances become very important. Consider swapping the multiplicand and multiplier when referring to a medication order:

- Give 3 milligrams of morphine 5 times per day
- Give 5 milligrams of morphine 3 times per day

In both these examples, the cumulative total, or product, is 15 milligrams of morphine given over a 24-hour period, but these two doses and administration schedules are drastically different.

The first step to multiplying is to memorize the multiplication table. In the multiplication table below, the multiplicand is represented in the vertical column on the left side of the table. The multiplier is across the top line, horizontally, on the table. By locating the intersection of the columns and lines represented by the multiplier and the multiplicand, you will find the correct answer.

For example, in the problem 9×7, 9 is the multiplier and 7 is the multiplicand. At the intersection of the two columns is the number 63, which is the product of the two numbers.

MULTIPLICATION TABLE

×	0	1	2	3	4	5	6	7	8	9	10	11	12
0	0	0	0	0	0	0	0	0	0	0	0	0	0
1	0	1	2	3	4	5	6	7	8	9	10	11	12
2	0	2	4	6	8	10	12	14	16	18	20	22	24
3	0	3	6	9	12	15	18	21	24	27	30	33	36
4	0	4	8	12	16	20	24	28	32	36	40	44	48
5	0	5	10	15	20	25	30	35	40	45	50	55	60
6	0	6	12	18	24	30	36	42	48	54	60	66	72
7	0	7	14	21	28	35	42	49	56	63	70	77	84
8	0	8	16	24	32	40	48	56	64	72	80	88	96
9	0	9	18	27	36	45	54	63	72	81	90	99	108
10	0	10	20	30	40	50	60	70	80	90	100	110	120
11	0	11	22	33	44	55	66	77	88	99	110	121	132
12	0	12	24	36	48	60	72	84	96	108	120	132	144

When multiplying whole numbers with more than one digit, it is easiest to set up the numbers in columns. For example:

176×87 becomes

$$
\begin{array}{r}
176 \\
\times\ 87 \\
\hline
\end{array}
$$

Multiply the digit in the ones column of the bottom number by each digit in the top number. Start by multiplying the 7 by 6 to get 42. Since 42 is greater than 9, you'll have to carry the 4.

$$
\begin{array}{r}
{}^{4}\\[-4pt]
176 \\
\times\ 87 \\
\hline
2 \\
\end{array}
$$

Multiply the 7 by 7 to get 49; add the carried 4 to get 53. Since 53 is greater than 9, you'll have to carry the 5.

$$
\begin{array}{r}
{}^{5\ 4}\\[-4pt]
176 \\
\times\ 87 \\
\hline
32 \\
\end{array}
$$

Multiply the 7 by 1 to get 7 and add the carried 5. The result, 12, is greater than 9, but there are no more digits to carry over, so just write down the 2 and then write the 1 down to the left.

$$
\begin{array}{r}
{\scriptstyle 5\ 4} \\
176 \\
\times\ 87 \\
\hline
1232
\end{array}
$$

Next, multiply the digit in the tens column of the bottom number by each digit of the top number, starting with $8 \times 6 = 48$. Write the 8 in the tens column. Since 48 is greater than 9, you'll have to carry the 4.

$$
\begin{array}{r}
{\scriptstyle 4} \\
176 \\
\times\ 87 \\
\hline
1232 \\
8
\end{array}
$$

Multiply the 8 by 7 to get 56 and add the carried 4 to get 60. Since 60 is greater than 9, you'll have to carry the 6.

$$
\begin{array}{r}
{\scriptstyle 6\ 4} \\
176 \\
\times\ 87 \\
\hline
1232 \\
08
\end{array}
$$

Multiply the 8 by 1 to get 8 and add the carried 6 to get 14. 14 is greater than 9, but there are no more digits to carry over, so just write down the 4 and then write the 1 to its left.

$$
\begin{array}{r}
{\scriptstyle 6\ 4} \\
176 \\
\times\ 87 \\
\hline
1232 \\
1408\ \
\end{array}
$$

Finally, add the bold numbers together to get the answer.

$$
\begin{array}{r}
176 \\
\times\ 87 \\
\hline
\mathbf{1232} \\
+\ \mathbf{1408}\ \ \\
\hline
15312
\end{array}
$$

The answer is 15,312.

Practice 3

1. $27 \times 12 =$

2. $134 \times 76 =$

3. $643 \times 81 =$

4. $129 \times 114 =$

5. $6,234 \times 276 =$

Division

Division is the inverse of multiplication. Think of division as splitting a number into equal parts. The number to be split into equal parts always comes before the division sign; it is referred to as the *dividend*. The number to the right of the division symbol is referred to as the *divisor*; it specifies how many times to split the dividend. The resulting answer is referred to as the *quotient*.

Consider the equation: $15 \div 5 = 3$

In the above equation, 15 is the dividend. The divisor asks you to split the dividend into 5 equal parts. When you split 15 into 5 equal parts, you get a quotient of 3.

$$15 \div 5 = 3$$

Dividend   Divisor   Quotient

Long division is the method generally preferred when solving problems without a calculator. This method is based on separating the problem into smaller parts to arrive at the correct answer. To correctly solve division problems, you must first be proficient in both multiplication and subtraction.

Example:

$462 \div 3 =$ _____

First, convert the problem to the long division format as shown below by placing the divisor (3) before the division bracket and placing the dividend (462) under it.

divisor ⟶ 3)462 ⟵ dividend

You can now begin to solve the problem by dividing one number at a time. The first number of the dividend is divided by the divisor, so 4 divided by 3 equals 1 with 1 remaining. Note that the 1 is placed on top of the division bracket. The 3 (1 × 3) is placed under the 4. The next step is to complete the subtraction step: 4 minus 3 equals 1.

```
    1
3)462
  3
  1
```

The next number to be divided, 6, is brought down, so the new number to be divided is 16. Thus, 16 has become the dividend.

```
    1
3)462
  3↓
  16
```

When 16 is divided by 3, the result is 5 with 1 again remaining. The 5 is placed next to the 1 on top of the division bracket, and 15 (5 × 3) is subtracted from 16.

```
   15
3)462
  3
  16
  15
   1
```

The next number, 2, is brought down, making the new number to be divided 12. Dividing 12 by 3 equals 4 with 0 remaining. The 4 is the last number to be placed on top of the division bracket.

```
  154
3)462
  3
  16
  15↓
   12
   12
    0
```

Therefore, the correct answer to the problem, or the quotient, is 154.

$462 \div 3 = 154$

The easiest method of checking your answer for accuracy is to reverse the process by multiplying the quotient by the divisor. The answer should be the same as the dividend.

```
 154   quotient
× 3    divisor
 462   divident
```

Unfortunately, long division problems (especially concerning medications) do not always work out to a whole number. Sometimes, numbers are left over. These are known as remainders. Here is an example of a problem with a remainder.

$436 \div 25 =$ _____

Remember, the first step is to set up the problem in long division format. In this example, the divisor is a two-digit number, making the problem slightly more difficult.

$25\overline{)436}$

Because the first number of the dividend, 4, cannot be divided by the divisor, 25, the first number of the quotient placed on top of the division bracket is 0. When the divisor is more than a single number, as it is in this problem, the quotient will often begin with one or more zeros, or those places may be left blank.

```
     0
25)436
    0
   ──
   43
```

Note that after subtracting the 0, the new number to be divided, or the new dividend, is 43.

```
    017
25)436
    0
   ──
   43
   25
   ──
   176
   175
   ───
     1
```

After completing the problem, there is a remainder of 1. The zero preceding the whole number is dropped, so 017 becomes 17. The correct answer to the problem is 17 with a remainder of 1. The letter *r* is sometimes used to express a remainder.

$436 \div 25 = 17$ r 1, or 17 remainder 1.

The remainder can also be expressed as a fraction by placing the remainder over the divisor.

$$436 \div 25 = 17\frac{1}{25}$$

Fractions will be covered in Chapter 2.

Practice 4

1. $198 \div 9 =$
2. $171 \div 3 =$
3. $845 \div 13 =$
4. $3{,}572 \div 76 =$
5. $9{,}856 \div 112 =$

ANSWERS AND EXPLANATIONS TO PRACTICE EXERCISES

Practice 1

1.   245

Begin by rewriting the problem with the numbers in a column. Remember to justify the numbers to the right. Add each column starting with the ones, then the tens, and so on. Remember to carry over to the next column as needed.

$$
\begin{array}{r}
147 \\
+\ 98 \\
\hline
245
\end{array}
$$

2.   1,059

Begin by rewriting the problem with the numbers in a column. Remember to justify the numbers to the right. Add each column starting with the ones, then the tens, and so on. Remember to carry over to the next column as needed.

$$
\begin{array}{r}
498 \\
+\ 561 \\
\hline
1,059
\end{array}
$$

3.   410

Begin by rewriting the problem with the numbers in a column. Remember to justify the numbers to the right. Add each column starting with the ones, then the tens, and so on. Remember to carry over to the next column as needed.

$$
\begin{array}{r}
326 \\
75 \\
+\ 9 \\
\hline
410
\end{array}
$$

4.   2,198

Begin by rewriting the problem with the numbers in a column. Remember to justify the numbers to the right. Add each column starting with the ones, then the tens, and so on. Remember to carry over to the next column as needed.

$$
\begin{array}{r}
1,362 \\
732 \\
89 \\
+\ 15 \\
\hline
2,198
\end{array}
$$

5.   3,310

Begin by rewriting the problem with the numbers in a column. Remember to justify the numbers to the right. Add each column starting with the ones, then the tens, and so on. Remember to carry over to the next column as needed.

$$
\begin{array}{r}
2,358 \\
863 \\
85 \\
+\ 4 \\
\hline
3,310
\end{array}
$$

Practice 2

1.   37

When subtracting numbers, remember to rewrite the problem in a column. Justify the columns to the right so that the ones and tens places line up. Begin by subtracting the ones, then the tens. Borrow from the next column to the left when the bottom number in the problem is larger than the top number.

$$
\begin{array}{r}
{\scriptstyle 4\ 14} \\
\cancel{54} \\
-\ 17 \\
\hline
37
\end{array}
$$

2. 253

When subtracting numbers, remember to rewrite the problem in a column. Justify the columns to the right so that the ones, tens, and hundreds places line up. Begin by subtracting the ones, then the tens, etc.

```
   296
 −  43
   253
```

3. 404

When subtracting numbers, remember to rewrite the problem in a column. Justify the columns to the right so that the ones, tens, and hundreds places line up. Begin by subtracting the ones, then the tens, etc. Borrow from the next column to the left when the bottom number in the problem is larger than the top number.

```
   1 10
   7₂0
 − 316
   404
```

4. 3,327

When subtracting numbers, remember to rewrite the problem in a column. Justify the columns to the right so that the ones, tens, hundreds, and thousands places line up. Begin by subtracting the ones, then the tens, etc.

```
   3,859
 −   532
   3,327
```

5. 4,389

When subtracting numbers, remember to rewrite the problem in a column. Justify the columns to the right so that the ones, tens, hundreds, and thousands places line up. Begin by subtracting the ones, then the tens, etc. Borrow from the next column to the left when the bottom number in the problem is larger than the top number.

```
   7  12 15 15
   8,365
 − 3,976
   4,389
```

Practice 3

1. 324

Begin by rewriting the problem in a column. Multiply the first digit (in the ones column) of the bottom number by each digit of the top number. Write the product under the line. Remember to carry numbers over if needed. Next, multiply the second number (tens column) by the entire top number. Write the product under the line, moving one place to the left. Add the products together for the correct answer.

```
     1
    27
  × 12
    54
    27
   324
```

2. 10,184

Begin by rewriting the problem in a column. Then multiply the top number by each digit in the bottom number. Add the two products together.

```
     134
   ×  76
     804
     938
  10,184
```

3. 52,083

Begin by rewriting the problem in a column. Then multiply the top number by each digit in the bottom number. Add the two products together.

```
    643
  ×  81
    643
  51 44
  52,083
```

4. 14,706

Begin by rewriting the problem in a column. Then multiply the top number by each digit in the bottom number. Add the two products together.

```
    129
  × 114
    516
   1 29
  12 9
  14,706
```

5. 1,720,584

Begin by rewriting the problem in a column. Then multiply the top number by each digit in the bottom number. Add the two products together.

```
   6234
  × 276
  37404
  43638
  12468
  1,720,584
```

Practice 4

1. 22

Convert the problem to the long division format by placing the divisor before the division bracket and the dividend under it. Solve the problem by dividing the number inside of the bracket, the dividend, by the number outside of the bracket, the divisor. Multiply each quotient by the divisor, and subtract the result as you solve the problem. The answer, or quotient, is written on top of the bracket.

```
      22
  9)198
   - 18
     18
   - 18
      0
```

2. 57

Convert the problem to the long division format by placing the divisor before the division bracket and the dividend under it. Then solve the problem.

```
      57
  3)171
   - 15
     21
   - 21
      0
```

3. 65

Convert the problem to the long division format by placing the divisor before the division bracket and the dividend under it. Then solve the problem.

```
       65
  13)845
    - 78
      65
    - 65
       0
```

4. 47

Convert the problem to the long division format by placing the divisor before the division bracket and the dividend under it. Then solve the problem.

$$
\begin{array}{r}
47 \\
76{\overline{\smash{\big)}\,3572}} \\
\underline{-\ 304} \\
532 \\
\underline{-\ 532} \\
0
\end{array}
$$

5. 88

Convert the problem to the long division format by placing the divisor before the division bracket and the dividend under it. Then solve the problem.

$$
\begin{array}{r}
88 \\
112{\overline{\smash{\big)}\,9856}} \\
\underline{-\ 896} \\
896 \\
\underline{-\ 896} \\
0
\end{array}
$$

CHAPTER QUIZ

Select the correct answer to each question.

1. $1{,}374 + 873 + 45 + 9 =$

   (A) 2,231   (C) 3,203

   (B) 1,233   (D) 2,301

2. $654 + 87 + 206 + 19 + 7 =$

   (A) 783   (C) 973

   (B) 884   (D) 1,063

3. $8{,}943 - 7{,}610 =$

   (A) 922   (C) 1,244

   (B) 1,333   (D) 2,111

4. $4{,}371 - 4{,}295 =$

   (A) 73   (C) 75

   (B) 74   (D) 76

5. $539 \times 77 =$

   (A) 41,503   (C) 32,604

   (B) 52,412   (D) 35,614

6. $883 \times 216 =$

   (A) 6,181   (C) 190,318

   (B) 87,947   (D) 190,728

7. $2,401 \times 15 =$

   (A) 25,225   (C) 36,015

   (B) 46,115   (D) 55,405

8. $275 \div 25 =$

   (A) 9   (C) 13

   (B) 11   (D) 15

9. $637 \div 49 =$

   (A) 9   (C) 16

   (B) 13   (B) 19

10. $1,440 \div 12 =$

    (A) 110   (C) 120

    (B) 112   (D) 122

ANSWERS AND EXPLANATIONS

1. D

Remember to align or justify all of the numbers to the right and set up the problem vertically.

2. C

Remember to align or justify all of the numbers to the right and set up the problem vertically.

3. B

Remember to set up the problem vertically before attempting to solve it.

4. D

Remember to set up the problem vertically before attempting to solve it.

5. A

First, set up the problem vertically. Second, multiply 539 by 7 and write the product under the line. Third, multiply 539 by 7 again and write the product under the line, moving it to the left one place value as shown. Add the two numbers together.

$$
\begin{array}{r}
539 \\
\times\ 77 \\
\hline
3773 \\
+\ 3773 \\
\hline
41{,}503
\end{array}
$$

6. D

First, set the problem up vertically. Second, multiply 883 by 6 and write the product under the line. Third, multiply 883 by 1 and write the product under the line, moving to the left one place value as shown. Fourth, multiply 883 by 2 and write the product under the line, moving to the left another place value as shown. Add the three numbers together.

$$
\begin{array}{r}
883 \\
\times\ 216 \\
\hline
5298 \\
883 \\
+\ 1766 \\
\hline
190{,}728
\end{array}
$$

7. C

First, set the problem up vertically. Second, multiply 2,401 by 5 and write the product under the line. Third, multiply 2,401 by 1 and write the product under the line, moving it to the left one place value as shown. Add the two numbers together.

$$
\begin{array}{r}
2401 \\
\times\ 15 \\
\hline
12005 \\
+\ 2401 \\
\hline
36{,}015
\end{array}
$$

8. B

Begin by setting up the problem vertically. Divide 27 by 25 and write the answer, 1, on top of the division bracket. Subtract 25 from 27. The difference is 2. Bring the 5 down and divide again. Dividing 25 by 25 gives 1. Write the 1 on top of the division bracket and subtract 25 from 25. The difference is 0. The correct answer is, therefore, 11.

```
       11
  25)275
   − 25
      25
    − 25
       0
```

9. B

Begin by setting up the problem vertically. Because the first number of the dividend, 6, cannot be divided by the divisor, 49, the first number of the quotient placed on top of the division bracket is 0, or this place may be left blank. Bring down the 3 and divide 63 by 49 and write the answer, 1, in the second place on top of the division bracket. Subtract 49 from 63. The difference is 14. Bring the 7 down and divide one more time. Dividing 147 by 49 gives 3. Write the 3 on top of the division bracket. The correct answer, therefore, is 13.

```
       13
  49)637
   − 0
      63
    − 49
      147
```

10. C

Begin by setting up the problem vertically. Divide 14 by 12 and write the answer, 1, on top of the division bracket. Subtract 12 from 14. The difference is 2. Bring the 4 down and divide again. Dividing 24 by 12 gives 2. Write the 2 on top of the division bracket, and subtract 24 from 24. The difference is zero. Bring the zero down and divide one more time. Zero divided by any number equals zero. The correct answer is, therefore, 120.

```
        120
  12)1440
    − 12
       24
     − 24
       00
     − 00
        0
```

CHAPTER 2

Fractions

Fractions tend to be a pretty intimidating concept, but if you take the time to understand what each part of a fraction represents, they become much easier to work with. The simplest definition of a fraction is: *part of a whole*. When it comes down to it, that's all a fraction such as $\frac{3}{4}$ represents. The tricky part is explaining what the *whole* is that you are taking parts of. Once you understand that, taking 3 parts from a whole that is split into 4 pieces makes a lot more sense.

UNDERSTANDING FRACTIONS

Let's start by referring to the whole that we're talking about as the denominator. The denominator, no matter what number it is, represents one *whole thing*. This is the bottom number of a fraction.

Think of the denominator as a pizza:

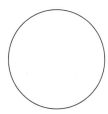

This is one whole pizza. It is one single piece. If this pizza represented our denominator, we would write it in terms of how many pieces it is composed of. In this case, just 1.

$$\overline{1}$$

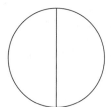

This is one whole pizza. The whole thing is still referred to as our denominator. The only difference here is that it has been split into 2 equal pieces. When referring to this whole pizza as our denominator, we write 2.

$$\overline{2}$$

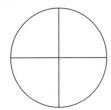

This is still one whole pizza. This pizza has been split into 4 equal pieces, or *parts*. When we write this whole pizza as a denominator, we write it as the number of equal pieces it's been split into.

$$\overline{4}$$

Look back at the three different pizzas above. The whole pizza that each of these three circles represents is exactly the same size; each one is just split up differently. That's all there is to a denominator. A denominator, no matter how big and ugly it may be, is nothing more than the number of equal pieces that make up one *whole thing*. That thing could be a pizza, a pill, or a bottle of water.

Now that you understand what a denominator represents, you've probably already figured out how the top number, the numerator, fits in. The numerator represents a given number of parts of the whole that you're dealing with.

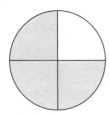

If we want to take 3 parts of a pizza that is made up of 4 equal pieces, remember that the denominator represents one whole pizza. The numerator specifies how many of those equal pieces, or parts, we want to take from the denominator.

$\underline{3}$ ← Numerator (number of pieces we want)
4 ← Denominator (number of pieces in the whole pizza)

TYPES OF FRACTIONS

There are four types of fractions:

1. **Common fractions** are those in which both the numerator and denominator are whole numbers, such as $\frac{3}{4}$.

2. In a **complex fraction,** the numerator and denominator are both fractions themselves, such as $\frac{\frac{1}{2}}{\frac{3}{4}}$. This type of fraction is not often used when calculating drug dosages.

3. **Proper fractions** are fractions in which the numerator is smaller than the denominator, such as $\frac{5}{8}$.

4. **Improper fractions,** such as $\frac{6}{4}$ or $\frac{8}{3}$, have a numerator that is larger than the denominator. An improper fraction can also be expressed as a **mixed number** (e.g., $\frac{6}{4} = 1\frac{2}{4}$ and $\frac{8}{3} = 2\frac{2}{3}$).

WORKING WITH FRACTIONS

When working with fractions, you will often need to do several things to complete a problem. Converting mixed numbers into improper fractions and improper fractions into mixed numbers, reducing fractions to their simplest forms (lowest terms), and finding a common denominator are important skills when calculating drug dosages.

Converting Fractions

Converting improper fractions into mixed numbers and converting mixed numbers into improper fractions is easy.

For example, convert $\frac{10}{3}$ to a mixed number.

> **STEP 1:** Divide the numerator (10) by the denominator (3). You will get 3 with 1 remaining.
>
> **STEP 2:** The 1 becomes the new numerator, and the denominator remains the same, 3.
>
> **STEP 3:** The mixed number is $3\frac{1}{3}$.

To convert a mixed number into an improper fraction, just reverse the process. We will use the answer to the example problem above, $3\frac{1}{3}$.

> **STEP 1:** Multiply the denominator (3) by the whole number (3). This equals 9.
>
> **STEP 2:** Add 9 to the numerator (1). This equals 10. The denominator remains the same, 3.
>
> **STEP 3:** The improper fraction is $\frac{10}{3}$.

Practice 1

1. Convert $\frac{5}{3}$ to a mixed number.

2. Convert $\frac{29}{24}$ to a mixed number.

3. Convert $5\frac{7}{8}$ to an improper fraction.

4. Convert $2\frac{4}{5}$ to an improper fraction.

> **Math Tip:** If your answers don't match those in the answer key, start by checking your basic arithmetic for errors.

Reducing Fractions

Reducing fractions makes them easier to understand. This means reducing both the numerator and the denominator to the smallest numbers possible.

For example, reduce the fraction $\frac{25}{100}$ to its lowest terms.

STEP 1: Determine the largest number by which both the numerator and denominator can be divided equally. Since they both end in 5, they are both multiples of 5. That means you can divide both numbers evenly by 5. (This doesn't work for all numbers but does work for numbers ending in 5.) In this case, the numerator and the denominator are divisible by both 5 and 25. Since 25 is larger, we will use that number to arrive at the final answer with the least number of steps.

STEP 2: Divide both the numerator and the denominator by the number determined in step 1 (25).

$25 \div 25 = 1$

$100 \div 25 = 4$

$\frac{25}{100}$ reduces to $\frac{1}{4}$.

STEP 3: Decide if the answer, $\frac{1}{4}$, can be reduced further. Determine if there is a number by which both the numerator and denominator can be divided equally. In this case, the numerator and the denominator are both divisible only by 1. Dividing by 1 will not change the numbers in the fraction, so this fraction is said to be in simplest form or lowest terms.

The fraction $\frac{25}{100}$ expressed in the simplest form or lowest terms is $\frac{1}{4}$.

> **Math Tip:** Not all fractions can be reduced. In the fraction $\frac{8}{13}$, the only number that both the numerator and the denominator can both be divided by is 1. Since dividing by 1 will not change the numbers in the fraction, this fraction is said to be in simplest form or lowest terms.

Practice 2

Reduce the following fractions to their simplest form or lowest terms.

1. $\frac{16}{24}$

2. $\frac{150}{500}$

3. $\frac{19}{21}$

Finding a Common Denominator

When adding and subtracting fractions, both fractions must have the same, or a common, denominator. While it is unlikely that you will have to add or subtract fractions with different denominators when calculating a drug dosage, the process is included in this chapter just in case you need a quick review.

For example, you need to perform addition or subtraction with the fractions $\frac{3}{5}$ and $\frac{7}{10}$.

> **STEP 1:** One of the easiest ways to find a common denominator is to multiply the denominators ($5 \times 10 = 50$). The common denominator for these fractions is 50.

> **STEP 2:** When the denominator is multiplied, the numerator must be multiplied as well. For $\frac{3}{5}$, the denominator was multiplied by 10, so the numerator must also be multiplied by 10 ($3 \times 10 = 30$). So $\frac{3}{5} = \frac{30}{50}$. You would need to complete the same process for $\frac{7}{10}$. Since the denominator was multiplied by 5, the numerator would also need to be multiplied by 5 ($7 \times 5 = 35$). So $\frac{7}{10} = \frac{35}{50}$.

Unfortunately, multiplying the denominators does not always result in the *lowest* common denominator. In the example above, the lowest common denominator of $\frac{3}{5}$ and $\frac{7}{10}$ is 10, not 50. By using the lowest common denominator, you work with smaller numbers and have less reducing to do at the end of solving the problem. Before beginning the problem, look at the denominators and determine the lowest number that can be divided into both without a remainder.

> **Math Tip:** In some cases, the lowest common denominator is the product of multiplying the denominators.

> **Math Tip:** If one of the fractions can be reduced, reduce it to its simplest form before attempting to determine the lowest common denominator.

Practice 3

Find the lowest common denominator for the following fractions.

1. $\frac{1}{3}$ and $\frac{5}{9}$

2. $\frac{1}{2}$ and $\frac{4}{9}$

3. $\frac{3}{5}$ and $\frac{5}{25}$

Adding and Subtracting Fractions

Now that you understand how to find the common denominator, adding fractions is simple.

Example: $\frac{3}{5} + \frac{7}{10} =$ _____

STEP 1: After finding the common denominator, add the numerators, or top numbers.

$\frac{6}{10} + \frac{7}{10} \Rightarrow 6 + 7 = 13$

STEP 2: Write the sum over the denominator, or bottom number.

$\frac{13}{10}$

STEP 3: If necessary, reduce the answer to its simplest form, or lowest terms. In this case, you will convert an improper fraction into a mixed number using the steps given earlier in this chapter and continue to reduce as needed.

$\frac{13}{10} = 1\frac{3}{10}$

So the answer to the example problem is $\frac{3}{5} + \frac{7}{10} = 1\frac{3}{10}$.

Subtracting fractions with a common denominator is just as easy as adding them.

Example: $\frac{5}{12} - \frac{1}{6} = $ _____

STEP 1: After finding the common denominator, subtract the numerators, or top numbers.

$$\frac{5}{12} - \frac{2}{12} \Rightarrow 5 - 2 = 3$$

STEP 2: Write the difference over the denominator, or bottom number.

$$\frac{3}{12}$$

STEP 3: If necessary, reduce the answer to its simplest form, or lowest terms.

$$\frac{3}{12} = \frac{1}{4}$$

So the answer to the example problem is $\frac{5}{12} - \frac{1}{6} = \frac{1}{4}$.

Practice 4

Solve the following addition and subtraction problems and reduce each answer to its lowest terms or simplest form.

1. $\frac{13}{18} + \frac{3}{5} =$

2. $\frac{1}{2} + \frac{5}{8} =$

3. $5 - \frac{7}{8} =$

4. $16\frac{3}{4} - 10\frac{5}{8} =$

> **Math Tip:** Pay close attention to the instructions when solving problems with fractions. If the instructions indicate that the answer should be expressed in its lowest terms or simplest form, failing to do so makes the answer incorrect. In the real world of dosage calculations, this is not commonly a problem.

Multiplying and Dividing Fractions

Multiplying and dividing fractions is even easier than adding and subtracting them, since there is no need to find a common denominator.

To multiply fractions, simply multiply the numerators and then multiply the denominators to find the product.

Example: $\frac{2}{3} \times \frac{3}{7} = $ _____

STEP 1: Set up the problem.

$$\frac{2 \times 3 =}{3 \times 7 =}$$

STEP 2: Multiply the numerators and then the denominators.

$$\frac{2 \times 3 = 6}{3 \times 7 = 21}$$

STEP 3: Determine if the answer, $\frac{6}{21}$, can be reduced. It can be reduced, so the correct answer is $\frac{2}{3} \times \frac{3}{7} = \frac{2}{7}$.

When dividing fractions, just as in multiplication, there is no need to find a common denominator. The most important step in dividing fractions is to set up the problem correctly.

Example: $\frac{2}{3} \div \frac{1}{4} = $ _____

STEP 1: Set up the problem. When dividing fractions, you must first invert the second fraction and then multiply the fractions.

$$\frac{2}{3} \div \frac{1}{4} = \frac{2}{3} \times \frac{4}{1}$$

STEP 2: Complete the multiplication.

$$\frac{2}{3} \times \frac{4}{1} = \frac{8}{3}$$

STEP 3: Reduce the answer to its lowest terms, in this case converting it from an improper fraction to a mixed number.

$$\frac{8}{3} = 2\frac{2}{3}$$

The answer to the example question is $\frac{2}{3} \div \frac{1}{4} = 2\frac{2}{3}$.

> **Math Tip:** The most important step in dividing fractions is to set up the problem correctly. Always invert the second fraction and then multiply straight across to get the correct answer.

To multiply or divide a fraction by a whole number, simply turn the whole number into a fraction by placing the whole number above the line and a 1 below it. For example, the whole number 2 expressed as a fraction is $\frac{2}{1}$, 7 is $\frac{7}{1}$, 12 is $\frac{12}{1}$, and so forth.

Example: $\frac{5}{16} \times 2 =$ _____

STEP 1: Turn the whole number 2 into a fraction.

$$2 = \frac{2}{1}$$

STEP 2: Set up the problem.

$$\frac{5}{16} \times \frac{2}{1}$$

STEP 3: Multiply the numerators and the denominators.

$$\frac{5}{16} \times \frac{2}{1} = \frac{10}{16}$$

STEP 4: Reduce the answer to its simplest form.

$$\frac{10}{16} = \frac{5}{8}$$

Practice 5

Solve the following multiplication and division problems and reduce the answers to their simplest form, or lowest terms.

1. $\frac{5}{8} \times \frac{5}{7} =$

2. $\frac{8}{9} \times \frac{3}{5} =$

3. $\frac{56}{100} \div \frac{4}{4} =$

4. $7 \div \frac{2}{3} =$

Converting Fractions to Decimals

Since most drug dosages and measuring devices use the metric system, you will need to be able to convert fractions to decimals. (Converting decimals to fractions will be covered in Chapter 3.)

Changing a common fraction into a decimal is easy if you follow a few simple steps.

Example: Convert $\frac{8}{16}$ into a decimal.

STEP 1: Divide the numerator by the denominator.

$8 \div 16 = .5$

STEP 2: Add a zero to the left of the decimal point to make the decimal point easier to see.

$.5 = 0.5$

So $\frac{8}{16} = 0.5$.

If you need to convert a mixed number into a decimal, you will need to turn the mixed number into an improper fraction first, then divide the numerator by the denominator. It is not necessary to add a zero to the left of the decimal point when a whole number is in that place.

Example: Convert $1\frac{1}{2}$ into a decimal.

STEP 1: Convert $1\frac{1}{2}$ into an improper fraction.

$1\frac{1}{2} = \frac{3}{2}$

STEP 2: Divide the numerator by the denominator.

$3 \div 2 = 1.5$

So $1\frac{1}{2} = 1.5$.

Practice 6

Convert the following fractions and mixed numbers into decimals.

1. $\frac{7}{8}$

2. $1\frac{3}{5}$

3. $12\frac{13}{14}$

ANSWERS AND EXPLANATIONS TO PRACTICE EXERCISES

Practice 1

1. $1\frac{2}{3}$

Divide the numerator (5) by the denominator (3). You will get 1 with 2 remaining. The 2 becomes the numerator, and the denominator remains the same (3). The correct answer is then $1\frac{2}{3}$.

2. $1\frac{5}{24}$

Divide the numerator (29) by the denominator (24). You will get 1 with 5 remaining. The 5 becomes the numerator, and the denominator remains the same (24). The correct answer is then $1\frac{5}{24}$.

3. $\frac{47}{8}$

Multiply the denominator (8) by the whole number (5). This equals 40. Add 40 to the current numerator, 7, to equal 47. The new numerator is 47; the denominator remains the same. The correct answer is $\frac{47}{8}$.

4. $\frac{14}{5}$

Multiply the denominator (5) by the whole number (2). This equals 10. Add 10 to the current numerator, 4, to equal 14. The new numerator is 14; the denominator remains the same. The correct answer is $\frac{14}{5}$.

Practice 2

1. $\frac{2}{3}$

Determine the largest number by which both the numerator and denominator can be divided equally. In this problem, both 16 and 24 are divisible by 8. Divide both the numerator and denominator by 8. The simplest form, or lowest terms, for this fraction is $\frac{2}{3}$.

$$\frac{16 \div 8 = 2}{24 \div 8 = 3}$$

2. $\frac{3}{10}$

Determine the largest number by which both the numerator and denominator can be divided equally. In this problem, both 150 and 500 are divisible by 50. Divide both the numerator and denominator by 50. The simplest form, or lowest terms, for this fraction is $\frac{3}{10}$.

$$\frac{150 \div 50 = 3}{500 \div 50 = 10}$$

3. $\frac{19}{21}$

There is no number that can be divided into both 19 and 21, so this fraction cannot be reduced further.

Practice 3

1. 9

In this problem, you have the option of multiplying the denominators to get a common denominator of 27. The lowest common denominator, however, is 9 because both 3 and 9, the denominators in the problem, can be divided into 9 without a remainder.

KAPLAN) NURSING

2. 18

The lowest common denominator for this problem is found by multiplying the denominators: $2 \times 9 = 18$.

3. 5

In this problem, $\frac{5}{25}$ can be reduced to $\frac{1}{5}$. Now both denominators are the same, so the lowest common denominator for this problem is 5.

Practice 4

1. $\frac{22}{15}$ or $1\frac{7}{15}$

The lowest common denominator for this problem is 15. The fraction $\frac{13}{15}$ remains the same. By multiplying both the numerator and the denominator in $\frac{3}{5}$ by 3, $\frac{3}{5}$ becomes $\frac{9}{15}$. You may now proceed with the addition.

$$\frac{13}{15} + \frac{9}{15} = \frac{22}{15}$$

Reduce $\frac{22}{15}$ to its lowest terms by dividing 22 by 15 to get 1 with a remainder of 7.

2. $1\frac{1}{8}$

The lowest common denominator for this problem is 8. The fraction $\frac{5}{8}$ remains the same. By multiplying both the numerator and the denominator in $\frac{1}{2}$ by 4, $\frac{1}{2}$ becomes $\frac{4}{8}$. You may now proceed with the addition.

$$\frac{4}{8} + \frac{5}{8} = \frac{9}{8}$$

Reduce $\frac{9}{8}$ to its lowest terms by dividing 9 by 8 to get 1 with a remainder of 1.

3. $4\frac{1}{8}$

Begin by turning the whole number 5 into a fraction, $\frac{5}{1}$. Next, find the common denominator. In this problem, it is easy; the common denominator is 8, since both 8 and 1 can be divided into 8 without a remainder. Multiple both the numerator and the denominator by 8.

$$\frac{5 \times 8 = 40}{1 \times 8 = 8}$$

The problem is now $\frac{40}{8} - \frac{7}{8}$. Simply subtract the second numerator from the first: $40 - 7 = 33$. Place the answer over the denominator and reduce it to its lowest term or simplest form: $\frac{33}{8} = 4\frac{1}{8}$.

4. $6\frac{1}{8}$

In this problem, you can ignore the whole numbers in the first step. Find the common denominator for $\frac{3}{4}$ and $\frac{5}{8}$. The common denominator is 8, so $\frac{3}{4}$ becomes $\frac{6}{8}$.

The problem is now $16\frac{6}{8} - 10\frac{5}{8}$. Subtract the whole numbers, then subtract the fractions.

$$16 - 10 = 6$$
$$\frac{6}{8} - \frac{5}{8} = \frac{1}{8}$$

The correct answer is $6\frac{1}{8}$.

Practice 5

1. $\frac{25}{56}$

Simply multiply the numerators and the denominators in this problem. Since $\frac{25}{56}$ cannot be reduced, it is the correct answer to the problem.

$$\frac{5 \times 5 = 25}{8 \times 7 = 56}$$

2. $\frac{8}{15}$

Simply multiply the numerators and the denominators in this problem.

$$\frac{8 \times 3 = 24}{9 \times 5 = 45}$$

Reduce the answer of $\frac{24}{45}$ to its lowest terms, or simplest form, by dividing the numerator and the denominator by 3. The correct answer is $\frac{8}{15}$.

3. $\frac{14}{25}$

To solve this problem, you must invert the second fraction. Note that both the numerator and the denominator in this problem are the same (4). To solve the problem, simply multiply the numerators and the denominators.

$$\frac{56 \times 4 = 224}{100 \times 4 = 400}$$

Reduce the answer $\frac{224}{400}$ to its lowest terms, or simplest form. The correct answer is $\frac{14}{25}$.

4. $10\frac{1}{2}$

Begin by turning the whole number 7 into a fraction, $\frac{7}{1}$. Invert the second fraction by changing $\frac{2}{3}$ into $\frac{3}{2}$. Set up the problem and multiply the numerators and denominators.

$$\frac{7 \times 3 = 21}{1 \times 2 = 2}$$

Remember to reduce the answer of $\frac{21}{2}$ to its lowest form by dividing 21 by 2. The correct answer is $10\frac{1}{2}$.

Practice 6

1. 0.875

Divide the numerator (7) by the denominator (8): $7 \div 8 = .875$. Add a zero to the left of the decimal point so that the correct answer is 0.875.

2. 1.6

Begin by turning the mixed number into an improper fraction: $1\frac{3}{5} = \frac{8}{5}$. Divide the numerator (8) by the denominator (5): $8 \div 5 = 1.6$. Since there is a whole number to the left of the decimal point, this is the final correct answer.

3. 12.928571

Begin by turning the mixed number into an improper fraction: $12\frac{13}{14} = \frac{181}{14}$. Divide the numerator (181) by the denominator (14): $181 \div 14 = 12.928571$. Since there is a whole number to the left of the decimal point, this is the final correct answer.

CHAPTER QUIZ

Solve each of the following problems and select the correct answer. Remember to reduce each solution to lowest terms before deciding on a final answer.

1. $\dfrac{3}{8} + \dfrac{5}{8} =$

    (A) 1   (C) $\dfrac{8}{16}$

    (B) $\dfrac{8}{8}$ (D) $\dfrac{1}{2}$

2. $\dfrac{9}{16} - \dfrac{1}{4} =$

    (A) $\dfrac{8}{12}$ (C) $\dfrac{5}{16}$

    (B) $\dfrac{9}{64}$ (D) $2\dfrac{1}{4}$

3. $1\dfrac{2}{3} + 6\dfrac{5}{6} =$

    (A) $5\dfrac{1}{6}$ (C) $7\dfrac{9}{6}$

    (B) $8\dfrac{1}{2}$ (D) $8\dfrac{3}{6}$

4. $5\dfrac{7}{9} - 5\dfrac{13}{18} =$

    (A) $\dfrac{1}{18}$ (C) $\dfrac{6}{18}$

    (B) $\dfrac{6}{9}$ (D) 0

5. $\dfrac{16}{25} \times \dfrac{3}{4} =$

    (A) $\dfrac{9}{29}$ (C) $\dfrac{64}{75}$

    (B) $\dfrac{48}{100}$ (D) $\dfrac{12}{25}$

6. $1\frac{1}{2} \times \frac{3}{4} =$

   (A) $\frac{9}{8}$ (C) $\frac{12}{6}$

   (B) $1\frac{1}{8}$ (D) 2

7. $2\frac{3}{4} \div \frac{4}{5} =$

   (A) $2\frac{4}{20}$ (C) $3\frac{7}{16}$

   (B) $2\frac{1}{5}$ (D) $3\frac{1}{2}$

8. $25 \div \frac{3}{4} =$

   (A) $\frac{100}{3}$ (C) $18\frac{3}{4}$

   (B) $\frac{75}{4}$ (D) $33\frac{1}{3}$

9. Convert $1\frac{3}{4}$ to a decimal.

   (A) 0.175   (C) 17.5

   (B) 1.75   (D) 175.0

10. Convert $\frac{2}{7}$ to a decimal.

    (A) 0.1415632   (C) 0.3509785

    (B) 0.2857142   (D) 0.5606126

ANSWERS AND EXPLANATIONS

1. A

In this problem, both fractions have the same denominator (8). Simply add the numerators (3 + 5 = 8) and place the sum of the numerators over the current denominator. This results in $\frac{8}{8}$. Remember to reduce the fraction, which becomes 1. The correct answer is then (A). Choice (B) is not correct because it has not been reduced.

2. C

The first step in solving this problem is to find a common denominator. Since both denominators, 16 and 4, are divisible by 4, the lowest common denominator that can be used here is 16. The first fraction remains unchanged at $\frac{9}{16}$. The second fraction $\frac{1}{4}$ becomes $\frac{4}{16}$. With both denominators the same, you may now subtract the second numerator from the first, resulting in a difference of 5. The correct answer is $\frac{5}{16}$, and this fraction cannot be reduced.

3. B

In this problem, you may begin by adding the whole numbers together first: 1 + 6 = 7. Because the denominators in the fractions are not the same, you must first find a common denominator and then add the fractions. In this problem, the lowest common denominator is 6. This means that $\frac{2}{3}$ becomes $\frac{4}{6}$ and $\frac{5}{6}$ remains unchanged. At this point, you can add the numerators together: 4 + 5 = 9. The sum of the fractions is $\frac{9}{6}$. This can be reduced to $1\frac{3}{6}$ and further reduced to $1\frac{1}{2}$. The last step requires you to add the sum of the whole numbers to the sum of the fractions: $7 + 1\frac{1}{2}$. The correct answer is $8\frac{1}{2}$.

4. A

You can tell by looking at this problem that the answer, or the difference, will be fairly small. Begin by finding the common denominator. In this problem, 18 can be used as the common denominator. This changes the first number to $5\frac{14}{18}$, and the second number remains unchanged. Begin by subtracting the numerator in the second fraction from the numerator in the first fraction: 14 − 13 = 1. Since the denominator does not change, the difference in the fractions is $\frac{1}{18}$. The whole numbers are easy: 5 − 5 = 0. That makes the correct answer to this problem $0 + \frac{1}{18}$, or $\frac{1}{18}$.

5. D

This problem is easy. Simply multiply the numerators: 16 × 3 = 48. Then multiply the denominators: 25 × 4 = 100. Write the numerator over the denominator: $\frac{48}{100}$. The trick here is to remember to reduce $\frac{48}{100}$ to its lowest terms, getting $\frac{12}{25}$. Choice (B) is incorrect because it was not reduced as the instructions indicated.

6. B

The first step in solving this problem is to convert $1\frac{1}{2}$ into an improper fraction: $1\frac{1}{2} = \frac{3}{2}$. Once you have converted the mixed number into a fraction, you may proceed with multiplying the numerators ($3 \times 3 = 9$) and the denominators ($2 \times 4 = 8$). Write the product of the numerators over the product of the denominators: $\frac{9}{8}$. Remember to reduce the answer to its lowest terms. If you forgot that step, you may have chosen (A) as the answer.

7. C

Begin by converting the mixed number $2\frac{4}{5}$ into the fraction $\frac{11}{5}$. Next, invert the second fraction so that $\frac{4}{5}$ becomes $\frac{5}{4}$. You can now simply multiply the numerators ($11 \times 5 = 55$) and the denominators ($4 \times 4 = 16$). Write the product of the numerators over the product of the denominators, and the initial answer is $\frac{55}{16}$. When this improper fraction is reduced to a mixed number, the answer is $3\frac{7}{16}$.

8. D

This problem is a little trickier. You have to remember to turn the whole number, 25, into the fraction $\frac{25}{1}$ before starting. After that point, it's simple. Invert the second fraction so that $\frac{3}{4}$ becomes $\frac{4}{3}$. Multiply the numerators ($25 \times 4 = 100$) and the denominators ($1 \times 3 = 3$). Write the product of the numerators over the product of the denominators and reduce it: $\frac{100}{3} = 33\frac{1}{3}$.

9. B

There is no need to make any changes to the whole number in this problem. The 1 remains unchanged. Working only with the fraction, divide 3 by 4. The answer is 0.75. Add the 1 and the 0.75 for a sum of 1.75. If you prefer to turn the mixed number into an improper fraction, you can work the problem that way as well. In this case, $1\frac{3}{4} = \frac{7}{4}$. Simply divide 7 by 4. The answer is still 1.75. The important part of solving this problem is to pay close attention to the location of the decimal point. If it is moved one place to the left or right, the answer is either $\frac{1}{10}$ as much or 10 times as much. The location of the decimal point is very important and will be covered in depth in Chapter 3.

10. B

Divide the numerator (2) by the denominator (7). The correct answer is 0.2857142. In most problems, you would have been instructed to round the answer to the nearest 10th or 100th. Rounding will be covered in Chapter 3. Since you were not instructed to round, the correct answer is (B).

Decimals

Imagine if intake and output, medications, and blood products were all measured as fractions, and that each of those fractions had different denominators. Before the move to metric, that's how things were measured in the hospital setting. Intake and output was measured in cups, pints, and quarts. Oral solutions were measured in teaspoons and tablespoons. IV fluids were measured in cubic centimeters (cc's), and blood products were measured in pints. Before all of these fluids could be added together or subtracted from one another, each had to be converted to a common unit. Converting each of those volumes to a common unit was a time-consuming and very error-prone process.

DECIMALS AND THE METRIC SYSTEM

The metric system, discussed in Chapter 7, is a system of measurement based on decimals. Rather than using fractions with different denominators, the decimal system is a way of representing numbers so that they always share a common denominator of 10, or a power of 10. For example, the decimal 0.9 represents $\frac{9}{10}$, or 9 tenths.

Numbers to the left of the decimal point are whole numbers that we are all familiar with. Each place to the left represents progressively larger numbers. With each step to the left, numbers increase by powers of 10 (e.g., 1, 10, 100, 1,000, etc.).

Numbers to the right of the decimal point have a value less than one and get progressively smaller. Each place to the right represents progressively smaller decimals. With each step to the right, decimals are divided by powers of 10 (e.g., 0.1, 0.01, 0.001, etc.).

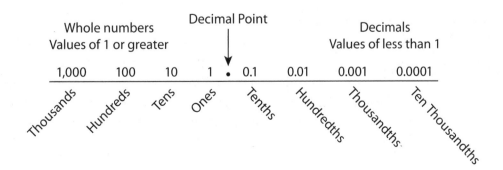

SPEAKING IN DECIMALS

When speaking a decimal, there are two different formats to choose from. The first is to read each number in sequence, including the decimal by saying "dot" or "point." The alternate pronunciation is to use labels to identify your decimal, in which case you would say "and" in place of the decimal point, followed by the label that corresponds to the last digit in the decimal. Here are a few examples:

Decimal		Pronunciations
100.7	→	"one hundred point seven" or "one hundred and seven tenths"
20.35	→	"twenty point three five" or "twenty and thirty-five hundredths"
1.225	→	"one point two two five" or "one and two hundred twenty-five thousandths"
0.5	→	"zero point five" or "five tenths"
0.01	→	"zero point zero one" or "one hundredth"

When pronouncing decimals with their corresponding label, there is no need to speak the leading zero, since you are appending a label at the end. When reading the digits aloud, however, it is good practice to always speak the leading zero.

For example: Saying "six tenths" is difficult to mistake for anything other than 0.6, but saying "point six" could easily be mistaken for "six" or even "twenty-six." Instead, say "zero point six."

AVOIDING DECIMAL ERRORS

To help prevent decimal errors, remember these two important rules:

1. **No trailing zeros.** A decimal should never end in a zero. Since a trailing zero is not expected in a decimal, a person could interpret a decimal that ends in zero as a whole number. For example: 2.50 can easily be mistaken for 250. Unlike a whole number, a decimal does not change its value when you remove a zero from the end. By dropping the zero, we don't change the value, but we decrease the likelihood of someone quickly assuming it's a whole number. The correct format for this decimal is: 2.5

2. **Decimals less than 1 *must* contain a leading zero.** When the value of a number is less than 1, always set a zero before the decimal. A decimal point should never be the first part of any number—it's too easily missed. For example: .45 can easily be mistaken for 45, especially if the decimal point is difficult to see. When a number is less than 1, always include a zero to the left of the decimal point. Whole numbers never begin with zeros, so this leading zero will quickly alert the reader to the decimal. The correct format for this decimal is: 0.45

Here are a few more examples:

Incorrect		Correct
18.50 (easily mistaken for 1850)	→	18.5
.5 (easily mistaken for 5)	→	0.5
1.80 (easily mistaken for 180)	→	1.8
.250 (easily mistaken for 250)	→	0.25

Practice 1

Write the following as decimal numbers.

1. Thirty-three hundredths

2. Two tenths

3. Four hundred seventeen thousandths

4. Sixteen hundredths

ADDING DECIMALS

Like whole numbers, decimal numbers may be added, subtracted, multiplied, and divided.

Decimal numbers are added using techniques similar to those used in adding whole numbers. The same math terminology is used.

STEP 1: Carefully write all decimal numbers in a column, aligning the decimal points directly beneath each other in a straight line. To make things easier, trailing zeros may be used to help keep the columns justified. For example (trailing zeros are in bold):

```
  12.100   (Two zeros are added to keep columns straight.)
   5.250   (One zero is added to keep columns straight.)
+  6.125
```

STEP 2: Bring the decimal point down to below the answer line.

```
  12.100
   5.250
 + 6.125
     .        (sum line)
```

STEP 3: Add the numbers in each column.

```
  12.100
   5.250
 + 6.125
  23.475
```

This answer is read as "twenty-three and four hundred seventy-five thousandths" or "twenty-three point four seven five."

Practice 2

1. 3.3 + 6.45 =

2. 15.6 + 1.47 + 5.03 =

3. 122.5 + 51.5 =

SUBTRACTING DECIMALS

To subtract decimal numbers, you will use techniques similar to those used in subtracting whole numbers. The same math terminology is used.

STEP 1: Write the decimals in a column, placing the decimal points directly beneath each other in a straight line. If you prefer, trailing zeros may be added to assist in keeping columns justified. For example: 11.33 – 6.15 = _____ becomes

```
  11.33
 - 6.15
```

And 3.25 – 2.98 = _____ becomes

```
  3.25
 - 2.98
```

STEP 2: Bring the decimal point down to below the difference or answer line. Subtract each column of numbers. For example:

```
  11.33
-  6.15
  5.18
```

The answer, or difference, is read as "five and eighteen hundredths" or "five point one eight."

```
  3.25
- 2.98
  0.27
```

If no whole number appears to the left of the decimal point, place a zero in the ones place, as shown above.

The difference is read as "twenty-seven hundredths" or "zero point two seven."

Practice 3

1. 17.5 – 6.12
2. 35.77 – 6.11

MULTIPLYING DECIMALS

Decimal numbers are multiplied in the same manner as whole numbers except for minor differences encountered in the final step. The same math terminology is used.

STEP 1: Write the problem with the greatest number of digits (multiplicand) above the number with the smaller number of digits (multiplier). For example:

```
  10.36  (multiplicand)
×  2.1   (multiplier)
```

STEP 2: Multiply the digit farthest to the right of the multiplier by each of the digits of the multiplicand. Carry numbers as necessary to the next place to the left. In this case, first multiply 1036 (the decimal point is not recognized until determining the final answer) by 1 and record the answer, as shown below.

$$
\begin{array}{r}
10.36 \\
\times\quad 2.1 \\
\hline
1036
\end{array} \leftarrow (1036 \times 1)
$$

STEP 3: Now multiply the next digit to the left in the multiplier (in this case 2) by 1036. This time, begin by placing the answer under the 3 and work to the left.

$$
\begin{array}{r}
10.36 \\
\times\quad 2.1 \\
\hline
1036 \\
2072\quad
\end{array}
\begin{array}{l}
\leftarrow (1036 \times 1) \\
\leftarrow (1036 \times 2)
\end{array}
$$

STEP 4: Add the columns.

$$
\begin{array}{r}
10.36 \\
\times\quad 2.1 \\
\hline
1036 \\
+\,2072\quad \\
\hline
21756
\end{array}
\begin{array}{l}
\text{(2 decimal places)} \\
\text{(1 decimal place)} \\
\leftarrow (1036 \times 1) \\
\leftarrow (1036 \times 2)
\end{array}
$$

STEP 5: Count the number of decimal places in both the multiplicand and the multiplier. In this problem, there are three.

STEP 6: In the answer, start from the right and count to the left the number of decimal places found in the problem (in this case three), and insert the decimal point. This is the final answer or product.

$$21757 \Rightarrow 21.756 \text{ (product)}$$

Practice 4

1. $22.5 \times 0.4 =$

2. $3.21 \times 1.5 =$

DIVIDING DECIMALS

When dividing decimal numbers, the equation should be set up as if you were dividing whole numbers. The same math terms are used.

STEP 1: Move the decimal point of the divisor to the end of the number, making it a whole number.

STEP 2: Move the decimal point in the dividend the same number of spaces as you moved the decimal point in the divisor.

For the following problem, the divisor has two decimal places, so 1.25 becomes 125 and 5.625 becomes 565.2.

5.652 ÷ 1.25 becomes $1.25\overline{)5.652}$, which becomes $125\overline{)565.2}$.

STEP 3: Place a decimal point in the quotient line directly above the decimal point in the dividend line.

$125\overset{\textstyle .}{\overline{)565.2}}$

STEP 4: Divide the numbers, adding zeros to the end of the dividend as needed.

125 goes into 565 four times. Put the 4 above the second 5.

```
        4.5216
125)565.2000    Note the addition of zeros to the dividend as needed.
    500         Multiply 125 by 4 (500) and subtract.
     65 2       125 goes into 652 five times. Put the 5 above the 2.
     62 5       Subtract 5 × 125 (625). Add a zero to the dividend; bring it down.
      2 70      125 goes into 270 two times. Place the 2 above the first zero.
      2 50      Subtract 2 × 125 (250). Add another zero to the dividend; bring it down.
        200     125 goes into 200 one time. Place the 1 above the second zero.
        125     Subtract 1 × 125 (125). Add a third zero to the dividend; bring it down.
        750     125 goes into 750 six times. Place the 6 above the third zero.
        750     Subtract 6 × 125 (750).
          0     The remainder is zero. Thus, the problem is finished.
```

The answer, or quotient, is 4.5216.

Math Tip: When the answer to a division problem contains infinite repeating numbers, this infinite repeating action is denoted by a series of periods (...) placed after at least three repeating numbers or a line over the numbers that repeat.

Practice 5

1. $6.5 \div 3.25 =$

2. $6.3 \div 1.5 =$

MULTIPLYING AND DIVIDING DECIMALS BY 10, 100, OR 1,000

Because doses in the metric system are expressed in values of 10, 100, 1,000, etc., converting doses in the metric system often is simply a matter of moving the decimal point.

Multiplying by 10, 100, or 1,000

To multiply, move the decimal point to the right. The number of zeros in the multiplier determines the number of places to move the decimal to the right, since we will be making the number larger. To multiply by 10, move the decimal one place to the right. To multiply by 100, move the decimal point to the right two places. To multiply by 1,000, move the decimal point to the right three places.

For example, to multiply 6.24 by 10, count the number of zeros. In this problem, there is one zero. You are making the number larger, so move the decimal point to the *right* one space, giving an answer of 62.4.

To multiply the same number by 100 (6.24 × 100), count the number of zeros. In this problem, there are two. Move the decimal point to the right two spaces, making the answer 624.

To multiply the same number by 1,000 (6.24 × 1,000), count the number of zeros. In this problem, there are three. Move the decimal point to the right three spaces. Because there is not a number after the 4, add a zero. This makes the answer 6,240.

Dividing by 10, 100, or 1,000

To divide a decimal number, move the decimal point to the left. The number of zeros in the divisor determines the number of places to move the decimal point. When dividing by 10, move the decimal point one place to the left. When dividing by 100, move the decimal point two places to the left. When dividing by 1,000, move the decimal place three places to the left.

For example, to divide 111.7 by 10, count the number of zeros. In this problem, there is one zero. Since we are making the number smaller, we move the decimal point to the *left* one place, giving an answer of 11.17.

To divide the same number by 100 (111.7 ÷ 100), move the decimal point to the left two places, making the answer 1.117. To divide the same number by 1,000, move the decimal point to the left three places. This makes our initial answer .1117, but because this could be misread, rewrite the final answer as 0.1117.

Practice 6

1. $1.019 \times 10 =$

2. $1.019 \times 100 =$

3. $1.019 \times 1,000 =$

4. $195.6 \div 10 =$

5. $195.6 \div 100 =$

6. $195.6 \div 1,000 =$

ROUNDING DECIMALS

Any number, including decimal numbers, may be rounded. When working with medications with a volume of 1 mL or greater, round to the tenths place. When the volume is less than 1 mL, it is rounded to the nearest hundredth.

STEP 1: Determine to which space the number should be rounded.

STEP 2: Look at the number immediately to the right of that number.

STEP 3: If the number immediately to the right of the number to be rounded is 4 or less, leave the number in the rounding place as is and drop all numbers to the right of it.

STEP 4: If the number behind the digit to be rounded is *5 or greater*, increase the digit in the rounding space by 1. Then drop all numbers to the right of it.

For example, round 0.657 to the hundredths place. The 5 is in the hundredths space, so look at the number to its right. In this problem, the number is 7. Therefore, the 5 is rounded up one digit, to 6, and all numbers to the right of it are dropped.

number place to round to (hundredths)

0.657 ◄——————— number that determines how rounding will be done

Therefore, the correct answer is 0.66.

Try another example: Round 2.43 to the nearest tenth. The tenths place is 4. Now look at the number to the right of the 4. That number, 3, is less than 5; therefore, the number in the rounding space is left as is, and all numbers to the right of it are dropped. The correct answer is 2.4.

Practice 7

Round questions 1 and 2 to the nearest tenth.

1. 11.89

2. 5.61

Round questions 3 and 4 to the nearest hundredth.

3. 0.955

4. 0.574

CONVERTING DECIMALS TO FRACTIONS

Changing decimals to fractions may be necessary when converting doses between two types of measurements. To do this, remove the decimal point and place the decimal number over whatever number is denoted by the place of the last digit.

Examples:

$$0.6 = \frac{6}{10}$$

$$0.25 = \frac{25}{100}$$

$$0.625 = \frac{625}{1,000}$$

Now reduce each fraction to its lowest form.

$$0.6 = \frac{6}{10} = \frac{3}{5}$$

$$0.25 = \frac{25}{100} = \frac{1}{4}$$

$$0.625 = \frac{625}{1,000} = \frac{125}{200} = \frac{5}{8}$$

Practice 8

Convert the following decimal numbers to fractions.

1. 0.8
2. 0.375

ANSWERS AND EXPLANATIONS TO PRACTICE EXERCISES

Practice 1

1. **0.33**
2. **0.2**
3. **0.417**
4. **0.16**

Practice 2

1. **9.75**

$$
\begin{array}{r}
3.3\mathbf{0} \\
+\ 6.45 \\
\hline
9.75
\end{array}
$$

Bring the decimal point down to the answer (sum) line. Starting in the column farthest to the right and working left, add the numbers as you would in a regular addition problem. The answer is read as "nine and seventy-five hundredths" or "nine point seven five."

2. **22.1**

$$
\begin{array}{r}
15.60 \\
1.47 \\
+\ 5.03 \\
\hline
22.1\cancel{0} = 22.1
\end{array}
$$

Bring the decimal point down to the answer (sum) line. Solve the problem as you would when subtracting whole numbers. Trailing zeros are deleted to get the final answer; the answer is read as "twenty-two and one tenth" or "twenty-two point one."

3. **174**

$$
\begin{array}{r}
122.5 \\
+\ 51.5 \\
\hline
174.\cancel{0} = 174
\end{array}
$$

Bring the decimal point down to the answer (sum) line. Add the numbers together. All trailing zeros are deleted, in this case leaving a whole number without any decimal numbers as the correct answer. The answer is read as "one hundred seventy-four."

Practice 3

1. **11.38**

$$
\begin{array}{r}
\overset{4\ 10}{17.5\cancel{0}} \\
-\ 6.12 \\
\hline
11.38
\end{array}
$$

Bring the decimal point down to the answer (difference) line. Subtract, remembering to borrow as necessary. The answer is read as "eleven and thirty-eight hundredths" or "eleven point three eight."

2. **29.66**

$$
\begin{array}{r}
\overset{2\ 15}{3\cancel{5}.77} \\
-\ 6.11 \\
\hline
29.66
\end{array}
$$

Bring the decimal point down to the answer (difference) line. Subtract, remembering to borrow when needed. The answer is read as "twenty-nine and sixty-six hundredths" or "twenty-nine point six six."

Practice 4

1. **9**

$$
\begin{array}{r}
\overset{1\ 2}{22.5} \\
\times\ 0.4 \\
\hline
900 \quad \leftarrow 225 \times 4 \\
+\ 000 \quad \leftarrow 225 \times 0 \\
\hline
\cancel{0}900 \rightarrow 9.\cancel{00} = 9
\end{array}
$$

Place the decimal point two places from the right and delete all trailing and unnecessary zeros.

2. **4.815**

$$
\begin{array}{r}
\overset{1}{3.21} \\
\times\ 1.5 \\
\hline
1605 \quad \leftarrow 321 \times 5 \\
+\ 321 \quad \leftarrow 321 \times 1 \\
\hline
4815 \rightarrow 4.815
\end{array}
$$

Place the decimal point three places from the right.

Practice 5

1. 2

$6.5 \div 3.25$ becomes $3.25\overline{)6.5}$

Move the decimal point in the divisor to the right until the divisor becomes a whole number. Now move the decimal point in the dividend the same number of places, adding zeros as needed. Place a decimal point in the quotient line directly above the decimal point in the dividend line.

Divide the dividend by the divisor, adding more zeros to the dividend as needed.

$$325\overline{)650.0}$$

325 goes into 650 two times. Place a 2 above the 0 immediately to the left of the decimal point.

$$\begin{array}{r} 2.0 \\ 325\overline{)650.0} \\ \underline{650} \quad \leftarrow 325 \times 2 \\ 0 \end{array}$$

The quotient, or answer, is 2.0 = 2 (trailing zeros are always deleted).

2. 4.2

$6.3 \div 1.5$ becomes $1.5\overline{)6.3}$

Move the decimal point in the divisor to the right until the divisor becomes a whole number. Now move the decimal point in the dividend the same number of places, adding zeros as needed. Place a decimal point in the quotient line directly above the decimal point in the dividend line.

$$15\overline{)63.0}$$

Divide the dividend by the divisor, adding zeros to the dividend as needed. The divisor, 15, goes into the dividend, 63, four times. Place a 4 on the quotient line above the 3.

$$\begin{array}{r} 4.2 \\ 15\overline{)63.0} \\ \underline{60} \\ 3\,0 \\ \underline{3\,0} \\ 0 \end{array}$$

60   Subtract 60 (4 × 15) and add a zero.

3 0   15 goes into 30 two times; place a 2 above the zero.

3 0   Subtract 30 (2 × 15) and bring down the zero.

0   When zero remains, the problem is solved.

The quotient, or answer, is 4.2.

Practice 6

1. 10.19

When multiplying by 10, the decimal is moved one place to the right.

2. 101.9

When multiplying by 100, the decimal is moved two places to the right.

3. 1,019

When multiplying by 1,000, the decimal is moved three places to the right.

4. 19.56

When dividing by 10, move the decimal point to the left one place.

5. 1.956

When dividing by 100, move the decimal point to the left two places.

6. 0.1956

When dividing by 1,000, move the decimal point to the left three places.

Practice 7

1. 11.9

Since the number to the right of the tenths place is greater than 5 (9), the 8 is rounded up to 9, and the 9 in the hundredths place is deleted, making the rounded answer 11.9.

2. 5.6

Since the number to the right of the tenths place is less than 5 (1), the 6 is left as is, and the 1 in the hundredths place is deleted, making the rounded answer 5.6.

3. 0.96

Since the number to the right of the hundredths place is 5 or greater (5), the 5 in the hundredths place is rounded up to 6, and the 5 in the hundredths place is deleted, making the rounded answer 0.96.

4. 0.57

Since the number to the right of the hundredths place is less than 5 (4), the 7 is left as is, and the 4 in the thousandths place is deleted, making the answer 0.57.

Practice 8

1. $\frac{4}{5}$

Delete the decimal point and place the 8 over 10 ($\frac{8}{10}$), because the 8 is in the tenths place. Now reduce the fraction to its lowest form.

2. $\frac{3}{8}$

Delete the decimal point and place the 375 over 1,000, because the digit farthest to the right in this number is in the thousandths place. Now reduce the fraction to its lowest form.

CHAPTER QUIZ

Solve each problem. Then select the correct answer.

1. Convert $\frac{7}{8}$ to decimal form.

    (A) 1.142857142   (C) 0.875

    (B) 0.88   (D) .88

2. Convert $\frac{5}{6}$ to decimal form.

    (A) 1.2   (C) .83

    (B) 0.833333…   (D) 0.83

3. $3.45 + 2.2 + 6.23 =$

    (A) 11.88   (C) 11.78

    (B) 12.98   (D) 12.88

4. $6.78 \times 1.7 =$

    (A) 11.5   (C) 1.1526

    (B) 115.26   (D) 11.526

5. $5.13 \times 6.6 =$

    (A) 3.385   (C) 0.338

    (B) 33.858   (D) 33.58

6. $10 \div 2.5 =$

    (A) 4   (C) 0.4

    (B) 4.0   (D) 40

7. $44 \div 2.2 =$

    (A) 2.20   (C) 2.0

    (B) 0.2   (D) 20

8. $1.83 \times 1,000 =$

    (A) 0.00183   (C) 1,830

    (B) 18.3   (D) 183

9. $35.44 \div 10 =$

    (A) 354.4   (C) 0.3544

    (B) 3.544   (D) 3,544

10. Round 123.986 to the nearest hundredth.

    (A) 123.9   (C) 123.986

    (B) 123.98   (D) 123.99

ANSWERS AND EXPLANATIONS

1. C

$7 \div 8 = 0.875$

2. B

$5 \div 6 = 0.8333\ldots$

3. A

```
  3.45
  2.20   (trailing zero added to help keep columns straight)
+ 6.23
─────
 11.88
```

4. D

```
    6.78
×   1.7
─────
   4746   ← 678 × 7
 + 678    ← 678 × 1
─────
  11526
```

The decimal point is placed three spaces from the right:

$11526 \to 11.526$.

5. B

```
    5.13
×   6.6
─────
   3078   ← 513 × 6
   3078   ← 513 × 6
─────
  33858
```

The decimal point is placed three spaces from the right:

$33858 \to 33.858$.

6. A

$2.5\overline{)10}$ becomes $25\overline{)100}$.

The divisor, 25, goes into 100 four times. Place a 4 above the second zero.

$$\begin{array}{r} 4. \\ 25\overline{)100} \\ \underline{100} \quad (4 \times 25) \\ 0 \qquad 0 \end{array}$$

When zero remains, the problem is solved. The answer is 4.

7. D

$44 \div 2.2$ becomes $2.2\overline{)44}$ becomes $22\overline{)440}$

The divisor, 22, goes into 44 two times. Place a 2 above the second 4 in the quotient line.

$$\begin{array}{r} 20. \\ 22\overline{)440} \\ \underline{44} \quad (2 \times 22) \\ 00 \\ \underline{0} \quad \text{22 goes into 0 zero times. Put a 0 in the quotient line above the 0.} \\ 0 \quad (22 \times 0) \end{array}$$

8. C

Move the decimal point three places to the right, adding zeros as necessary to get 1,830.

9. B

Move the decimal point one place to the left to get 3.544.

10. D

Because the number in the thousandths place is 5 or greater (6), the number in the hundredths place is rounded up, making the final rounded answer 123.99.

CHAPTER 4

Percentages

Percent means "parts per 100." In place of the word *percent*, percentages are often denoted by appending a percent sign (%). For example, the value 25% is read as "twenty-five percent" and interpreted as 25 parts per 100. Consider the grid below:

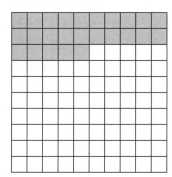

The shaded area represents 25 parts per 100, or 25%.

This value can also be expressed as a fraction: $\frac{25}{100}$.

Since a percent is always in the form of parts per 100, a percent can also be expressed as a decimal. The shaded area represents twenty-five hundredths, or 0.25.

In health care, percentages are often used to identify the strength of medications. For example, a solution of 50% dextrose in water contains 50% dextrose, while the other 50% is water. A tube of 2% hydrocortisone ointment contains 2 parts hydrocortisone, while the other 98 parts consist of oil, minerals, and other inactive ingredients.

As you can see from the diagram above, any percent can be converted to a fraction, and any fraction can be converted to a percent. A percent is also easily converted to a decimal, and a decimal to a percent. In this chapter, you will have an opportunity to become familiar with each of these conversions before using them in Chapter 5: Ratios and Proportions.

CONVERTING A PERCENT TO A FRACTION

To perform this type of conversion, first write the percent number (without the percent sign) as the numerator of a fraction. Now write 100 as the denominator. The final step is to reduce the fraction to its lowest form, or common terms.

For example, 15% becomes $\frac{15}{100}$. After the fraction is reduced (in this case, divide both the numerator and denominator by 5), the final answer is $\frac{3}{20}$.

In another example, 42% becomes $\frac{42}{100}$. After the fraction is reduced (in this case, divide both the numerator and denominator by 2), the final answer is $\frac{21}{50}$.

Practice 1

Convert each percent to its equivalent fraction form.

1. 75%
2. 99%
3. 12%
4. 6%

CONVERTING A FRACTION TO A PERCENT

First, convert the fraction to a decimal number. Now round the decimal number to the nearest hundredth. Then convert the decimal number to a percent.

For example, convert $\frac{3}{4}$ to a decimal by dividing 3 by 4: $3 \div 4 = 0.75$. There are two ways to complete the next step. The first choice is to move the decimal point to the right two places and add the percent sign to get 75%. The second choice is to multiply 0.75 by 100 ($0.75 \times 100 = 75$) and add the percent sign to make 75%.

In another example, convert $\frac{3}{8}$ to a decimal by dividing 3 by 8: $3 \div 8 = 0.375$. There are two ways to complete the next step. The first choice is to move the decimal point to the right two places and add the percent sign to get 37.5%. The second choice is to multiply 0.375 by 100 ($0.375 \times 100 = 37.5$) and add the percent sign to make 37.5%.

Practice 2

Convert each fraction to a percent.

1. $\dfrac{9}{10}$

2. $\dfrac{2}{3}$

3. $\dfrac{2}{5}$

4. $\dfrac{4}{5}$

CONVERTING A PERCENT TO A DECIMAL

Changing a percent to a decimal number can be an easy task. The first step is to remove the percent sign. The next step is as simple as dividing by 100 or moving the decimal point to the left two places.

For example, convert 65% to a decimal.

First, remove the percent sign to get 65. Use your method of choice to solve this problem.

1. Divide by 100: $65 \div 100 = 0.65$ (remember always to add a zero to the left of the decimal point when there is no whole number).

2. Move the decimal point to the left two places: 65 becomes 0.65.

For another example, convert $\frac{1}{4}$ percent to a decimal.

1. For this problem, first convert $\frac{1}{4}$ to a decimal number. Do this by dividing 1 by 4: $1 \div 4 = 0.25$. Now add the percent sign and get the decimal equivalent, 0.25%. Remove the percent sign and divide 0.25 by 100: $0.25 \div 100 = 0.0025$.

2. Make the same fraction-to-decimal conversion by moving the decimal point two places to the left, adding zeros as necessary: 0.25 becomes 0.0025.

Practice 3

Convert each percent to a decimal equivalent.

1. 29%

2. 18%

3. 59%

4. 34%

CONVERTING A DECIMAL TO A PERCENT

Some situations may require the nurse to convert decimals to percents. Multiplying by 100 easily accomplishes this task. To convert a decimal to a percent, multiply the decimal by 100 or move the decimal point two places to the right. Then add the % symbol to the last digit on the right of that number.

For example, convert 0.001 to a percent. You can choose from two methods to calculate this problem.

1. Multiply 0.001 by 100: $0.001 \times 100 = 0.1$. Then add the percent symbol to get 0.1%.

2. Move the decimal point to the right two places: 0.001 becomes 0.1. Then add the percent symbol to get 0.1%.

Sometimes when converting a decimal to a percent, it is necessary to add zeros to get the correct answer.

For example, convert 0.3 to a percent. Using your method of choice, calculate this problem.

1. Multiply 0.3 by 100: $0.3 \times 100 = 30$ (add a zero to obtain the correct answer). Then add the percent symbol to get 30%.

2. Move the decimal point to the right two places: 0.3 becomes 30 (again, add a zero to obtain the correct answer). Then add the percent symbol to get 30%.

Practice 4

Convert the following decimals to percents.

1. 0.004

2. 0.85

3. 0.1

4. 0.125

PERCENT USAGE IN SOLUTIONS AND MEDICATIONS

Percentage is frequently used to denote the strength of a liquid medication, ointment, or solution. A *solution* is a liquid mixture that contains a certain amount of solute and the diluent to which the solute is added. The *percent strength* of the solution is the amount of solute that is found in 100 mL of solution. The higher the percentage on the drug labels, the higher the strength of the solution or drug.

For example, a 5 percent solution always has a higher strength than a 2.5 percent solution.

5% solution

2.5% solution

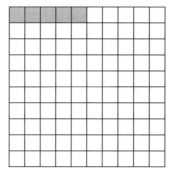
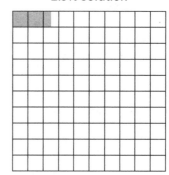

Practice 5

In each of the following pairs of percentages, identify the higher-strength doses.

1. 0.1% or 1%

2. 2.5% or 0.25%

3. 0.3% or 0.25%

4. 0.01% or 0.3%

ANSWERS AND EXPLANATIONS TO PRACTICE EXERCISES

Practice 1

1. $\frac{3}{4}$

Change 75% to $\frac{75}{100}$ and reduce.

2. $\frac{99}{100}$

Change 99% to $\frac{99}{100}$. This fraction is already in its lowest form, or common terms.

3. $\frac{3}{25}$

Change 12% to $\frac{12}{100}$ and reduce.

4. $\frac{3}{50}$

Change 6% to $\frac{6}{100}$ and reduce.

Practice 2

1. 90%

Convert $\frac{9}{10}$ to a decimal by dividing 9 by 10: $9 \div 10 = 0.9$. There are two ways to complete the next step. One method is to move the decimal point to the right and add a necessary zero. The other way is to multiply 0.9 by 100 ($0.9 \times 100 = 90$). Either way, the final step is to add the percent sign.

2. 67%

Convert $\frac{2}{3}$ to a decimal by dividing 2 by 3: $2 \div 3 = 0.666$. Round this number to the nearest hundredth to get 0.67. There are two ways to complete the next step. One is to move the decimal point to the right. The other is to multiply 0.67 by 100 ($0.67 \times 100 = 67$). Either way, the final step is to add the percent sign.

3. 40%

Convert $\frac{2}{5}$ to a decimal by dividing 2 by 5: $2 \div 5 = 0.4$. There are two ways to complete the next step. One method is to move the decimal point to the right and add the necessary zero to get 40. The other method is to multiply 0.4 by 100 ($0.4 \times 100 = 40$). Either way, the final step is to add the percent sign.

4. 80%

Convert $\frac{4}{5}$ to a decimal by dividing 4 by 5: $4 \div 5 = 0.8$. There are two ways to complete the next step. One is to move the decimal point to the right and add the necessary zero to get 80. The other choice is to multiply 0.8 by 100 ($0.8 \times 100 = 80$). Either way, the final step is to add the percent sign.

Practice 3

1. 0.29

Remove the percent sign and divide by 100: $29 \div 100 = 0.29$. (Remember to place a zero in the ones place when the answer is less than 1.) Or remove the percent sign (29% becomes 29) and move the decimal point two places to the left (29 becomes 0.29).

2. 0.18

Remove the percent sign and divide by 100: $18 \div 100 = 0.18$. (Remember to place a zero in the ones place when the answer is less than 1.) Or remove the percent sign (18% becomes 18) and move the decimal point two places to the left (18 becomes 0.18).

3. 0.59

Remove the percent sign and divide by 100: $59 \div 100 = 0.59$. (Remember to place a zero in the ones place when the answer is less than 1.) Or remove the percent sign (59% becomes 59) and move the decimal point two places to the left (59 becomes 0.59).

4. 0.34

Remove the percent sign and divide by 100: $34 \div 100 = 0.34$. (Remember to place a zero in the ones place when the answer is less than 1.) Or remove the percent sign (34% becomes 34) and move the decimal point two places to the left (34 becomes 0.34).

Practice 4

1. $0.004 \times 100 = 0.4\%$

Move the decimal point to the right two spaces, and 0.004 becomes 0.4. Then add the percent sign.

2. $0.85 \times 100 = 85\%$

Move the decimal point to the right two spaces, and 0.85 becomes 85. Then add the percent sign.

3. $0.1 \times 100 = 10\%$

Move the decimal point to the right two spaces, and 0.1 becomes 10 (adding one zero on the right). Then add the percent sign.

4. $0.125 \times 100 = 12.5\%$

Move the decimal point to the right two spaces, and 0.125 becomes 12.5. Then add the percent sign.

Practice 5

1. **1%**

2. **2.5%**

3. **0.3%**

4. **0.3%**

CHAPTER QUIZ

Solve each problem. Then select the correct answer. Remember to reduce each solution to lowest terms.

1. Convert 0.005 to a percent.

   (A) .5%   (C) 50%
   (B) 0.5%   (D) 0.05%

2. Convert 0.4 to a percent.

   (A) .4%   (C) 40%
   (B) 0.4%   (D) 0.04%

3. Convert 10% to a decimal.

   (A) 0.1   (C) 100
   (B) 10   (D) 0.01

4. Convert 50% to a fraction.

   (A) $\frac{50}{100}$ (C) $\frac{1}{2}$
   (B) $\frac{5}{10}$ (D) $\frac{2}{1}$

5. Convert $\frac{6}{10}$ to a percent.

   (A) 600%   (C) 6%
   (B) 0.6%   (D) 60%

6. Convert $\frac{3}{15}$ to a percent.

    (A) 20%   (C) 0.2%

    (B) 2%   (D) 200%

7. Identify the higher strength dose, 0.5% or 0.25%.

    (A) 0.5%   (B) 0.25%

8. Identify the higher strength dose, 0.4% or 0.04%.

    (A) 0.4%   (B) 0.04%

9. Convert $\frac{7}{21}$ to a percent.

    (A) 3%   (C) 0.3%

    (B) 33%   (D) 0.33%

10. Convert 1.35 to a percent.

    (A) 1.35%   (C) 135%

    (B) 13.5%   (D) 0.135%

ANSWERS AND EXPLANATIONS

1. B

$0.005 \times 100 = 0.5\%$

Or move the decimal point to the right two places to get 0.5%.

2. C

$0.4 \times 100 = 40\%$

Or move the decimal point to the right two places to get 40%.

3. A

Remove the percent sign and divide 10 by 100 to get 0.1, or remove the percent sign and move the decimal to the left two places to get 0.1.

4. C

Place 50 over 100 to get $\frac{50}{100}$ and reduce the fraction to its lowest form, or common terms, to get $\frac{1}{2}$.

5. D

$6 \div 10 = 0.6$

Then either move the decimal point to the right two places and add the percent sign to get 60%, or multiply 0.6 by 100 to get 60 and then add the percent sign to get 60%.

6.   A

$3 \div 15 = 0.2$

Then either move the decimal point to the right two places and add the percent sign to get 20%, or multiply 0.2 by 100 to get 20 and then add the percent sign to get 20%.

7.   A

The number 0.5% is higher than 0.25% and, therefore, the higher dose.

8.   A

The number 0.4% is higher than 0.04% and, therefore, the higher dose.

9.   B

$7 \div 21 = 0.333\ldots$

Round to the hundredth to get 0.33. Then either move the decimal point to the right two places and add the percent sign to get 33%, or multiply 0.33 by 100 to get 33 and then add the percent sign to get 33%.

10.   C

$1.35 \times 100 = 135\%$

Or move the decimal point to the right two places to get 135%.

Ratios and Proportions

Now that you have a good understanding of fractions, decimals, and percentages, it is time to move on to ratios and proportions. Ratios and proportions are methods used to calculate medication dosages. A ratio may be used to describe the quantity of a liquid drug in proportion to the solution it is in, such as with IV medications. Using ratios and proportions helps nurses to determine how many tablets of a specific medication to give when the dose ordered is more than one tablet.

Chapter 5 covers the process for converting ratios into fractions, decimals, percentages, and back into ratios. It also explains how to check a proportion equation to determine if it is true and equal and solve for the variable *x*. Using ratios and proportions to solve dosage calculation problems will be covered in Chapter 8: Basic Problem Solving and Strategies for Dosage Calculation.

UNDERSTANDING RATIOS

In terms of dosage calculation, ratios are treated like fractions. Just as the numerator referred to part of the denominator, a ratio shows the relationship of a particular part to a whole. In a ratio, the two numbers are separated by a colon (:) instead of a fraction bar (—).

Consider the following grid:

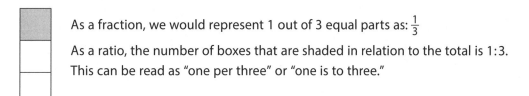

As a fraction, we would represent 1 out of 3 equal parts as: $\frac{1}{3}$

As a ratio, the number of boxes that are shaded in relation to the total is 1:3. This can be read as "one per three" or "one is to three."

Now consider the following grids:

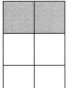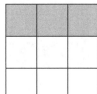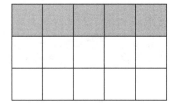

Each of the grids above represents a different fraction $\left(\frac{2}{6}, \frac{3}{9}, \frac{5}{15}\right)$, but each reduces to the same fraction: $\frac{1}{3}$. So, we could say that each grid represents a ratio of 1:3. Each column above is identical to the next and represents a ratio of 1:3. We can repeat the columns indefinitely, and although the number of columns goes up incrementally, the ratio stays the same.

CONVERTING FRACTIONS INTO RATIOS

It is easy to convert ratios to fractions as well as to convert fractions to ratios.

Examples:

$$1:2 = \frac{1}{2}$$

$$5:8 = \frac{5}{8}$$

$$\frac{7}{16} = 7:16$$

$$\frac{3}{5} = 3:5$$

> **Math Tip:** When converting between ratios and fractions, no calculations are necessary. Simply change the way the numbers are presented.

Ratios, like fractions, are usually expressed in their lowest terms or simplest forms. For example, the fraction $\frac{10}{50}$ would be reduced to $\frac{1}{5}$. Likewise, the ratio 10:50 should be expressed by reducing it to 1:5.

> **Math Tip:** Chapter 2 covered the steps required to reduce fractions. Go back and review if you are unsure of the correct way to reduce fractions.

CONVERTING DECIMALS INTO RATIOS

Decimals can be converted easily into ratios, and ratios converted into decimals just as easily. Follow the steps to convert a ratio to a decimal in the following example.

Convert 3:10 into a decimal.

STEP 1: Write the ratio as a fraction: 3:10 becomes $\frac{3}{10}$.

STEP 2: Convert the fraction to a decimal by dividing the numerator by the denominator: $3 \div 10 = 0.3$. Therefore, $3:10 = \frac{3}{10} = 0.3$.

To convert a decimal to a ratio, just reverse the process.

For example, convert 0.25 to a ratio.

STEP 1: Write the decimal as a fraction: $0.25 = \frac{25}{100}$.

STEP 2: Reduce the fraction to lowest terms: $\frac{25}{100} = \frac{1}{4}$.

STEP 3: State the fraction as a ratio: $\frac{1}{4} = 1:4$.

CONVERTING PERCENTAGES INTO RATIOS

Percentages can also be converted into ratios and ratios into percentages. Remember that a percentage is simply a fraction with a denominator of 100: 25 percent is the same as $\frac{25}{100}$, and 12 percent is the same as $\frac{12}{100}$. The following steps will help you work through the process of converting ratios and percentages.

> **Math Tip:** Go back and review Chapter 4 if you need additional help converting percentages into fractions.

For example, convert the ratio 2:25 into a percent.

STEP 1: Convert the ratio into a decimal: $2:25 = 2 \div 25 = 0.08$.

STEP 2: Multiply 0.08 by 100 and add the percent symbol: $0.08 \times 100 = 8\%$.

For another example, convert 22 percent into a ratio.

STEP 1: Write the percent as a fraction: $22\% = \frac{22}{100}$.

STEP 2: Reduce the fraction to its lowest terms: $\frac{22}{100} = \frac{11}{50}$.

STEP 3: State the fraction as a ratio: $\frac{11}{50} = 11:50$.

Practice 1

1. Convert the ratio 3:7 to a fraction.

2. Convert the fraction $\frac{11}{12}$ to a ratio.

3. Convert the decimal 0.67 to a ratio.

4. Convert the ratio 3:2 to a decimal.

5. Convert the ratio 2:9 to a percent. If necessary, round to the nearest percent.

6. Convert 400% to a ratio.

LOOKING AT PROPORTIONS

A proportion is simply two or more ratios that are equal. Consider two of the example grids from the beginning of the chapter. If we did not reduce their ratios to lowest common terms, they would correlate as follows:

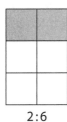   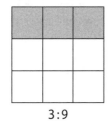

2:6   3:9

Knowing that both of the above ratios reduce to the same lowest common ratio (1:3), we can say that they are equal, or equivalent, to one another. When writing proportions, a double colon (::) is often used in place of an equal sign.

There are several ways to write this proportion:

$\frac{2}{6} = \frac{3}{9}$ shows the two fractions separated by an equal sign.

2:6 = 3:9 shows the two ratios separated by an equal sign.

2:6 :: 3:9 shows the two ratios separated by a double colon.

Remember that when reading a ratio, the single colon is read as "is to" or "per." The double colon in a proportion is read as "as." The proportion above would be read as: "two is to six as three is to nine."

Converting fraction proportions to ratio-proportions requires two simple steps, as shown in this example.

Write the fraction proportion $\frac{2}{7} = \frac{6}{21}$ as a ratio-proportion.

STEP 1: Convert each fraction to a ratio.

$\frac{2}{7}$ becomes 2:7, and $\frac{6}{21}$ becomes 6:21, so 2:7 = 6:21

STEP 2: Replace the equal sign (=) with a double colon (::).

2:7 :: 6:21

Converting a ratio-proportion to a fraction proportion just uses the opposite process.

For example, write the ratio-proportion 4:3 :: 20:15 as a fraction proportion.

STEP 1: Replace the double colon (::) with an equal sign (=).

4:3 = 20:15

STEP 2: Convert both ratios to fractions.

$\frac{4}{3} = \frac{20}{15}$

There is an easy way to determine if a proportion equation is correct and the ratios are equal. The terms in a proportion have specific mathematical names. The numbers in the middle of the equation are referred to as the *means*. The numbers on the outside or on the ends of the equations are called the *extremes*.

Let's look again at the example of 1:3 :: 3:9.

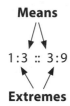

Means

1:3 :: 3:9

Extremes

Math Tip: An easy way to remember the terms is to note that *means* begins with the letter *m*, as does the word *middle*. The means are in the middle. *Extremes* begins with the letter *e*, as does the word *end*. The extremes are on the ends.

To determine if an equation is true and equal, simply multiply the means and then multiply the extremes. In this case:

Means: $3 \times 3 = 9$
Extremes: $1 \times 9 = 9$

The products should be the same. If they are not, the equation is not true and equal.

> **Math Tip:** In a proportion equation, the product of the means equals the product of the extremes.

Here is another example:

6:1 :: 12:2

This would be read as, "Six is to one as twelve is to two."

To determine if this equation is true and equal, first multiply the means (middle numbers).

$1 \times 12 = 12$

Next, multiply the extremes (end numbers).

$6 \times 2 = 12$

If the product of the means equals the product of the extremes, the equation is correct.

This skill is very important when checking your calculations prior to administering a medication. With that in mind, let's move on to solving an equation when it is missing one of the means or one of the extremes. This is commonly called "solving for *x*."

Practice 2

1. Write the fraction proportion $\frac{8}{9} = \frac{16}{18}$ as a ratio-proportion.

2. Write the ratio-proportion 50:75 :: 100:150 as a fraction proportion.

3. Is the proportion 6:7 :: 12:15 true and equal?

4. Is the proportion 7:4 :: 21:12 true and equal?

SOLVING FOR *X*

Solving for the variable *x* is used when solving an equation in which three of the numbers in the ratios are known and one is not. The *x* represents the fourth number or the part of the equation that is unknown.

Because the product of the means is always equal to the product of the extremes, it is easy to solve an equation in which you know three of the numbers.

For example, solve for *x* in the following equation.

$3:4::x:12$

STEP 1: Multiply the means and the extremes.

$4 \times x = 4x$ (means)
$3 \times 12 = 36$ (extremes)

Therefore:

$4x = 36$

STEP 2: Divide both sides of the equation by the number in front of the *x*, 4.

$4x \div 4 = x$
$36 \div 4 = 9$
$x = 9$

To help you better understand the concept, we will do a simple problem involving the purchase of apples. Earlier in the chapter, we used an example of 1 *is to* 3 *as* 3 *is to* 9; we'll continue to use those numbers. Suppose you went to the market and a sign in the produce aisle indicated that apples were on sale, 3 for $1. Your favorite pie recipe calls for 9 apples. How much would 9 apples cost?

You have three of the numbers necessary to set up this problem as a proportion.

It costs $1 for 3 apples, so $1 is to 3 apples as *x* is to 9 apples.

The equation would look like this:

$1:3::x:9$

To determine how much 9 apples would cost, you would need to solve for *x*. To do this, begin by multiplying the means: $3 \times x = 3x$. Then multiply the extremes: $1 \times 9 = 9$.

For the equation to be true and equal, the product of the means and the extremes must be the same. In other words, $9 = 3x$.

Divide both sides of the equation by the number in front of the *x*, in this case 3.

$$\frac{9}{3} = \frac{3x}{3}$$
$$3 = x$$

It would cost $3 to buy 9 apples.

> **Math Tip:** Pay attention when setting up the equation. If the first number on the left side of the equation represents apples, the first number must also represent apples on the right side of the equation. If the second number on the left side of the equation represents dollars, it must also represent dollars on the right side. Failing to follow this simple rule will result in an incorrect answer.

Solving for *x* in a fraction proportion can be done by cross multiplying. You are basically completing the same process; it is just written in a different format.

For example, solve for *x* in the following fraction proportion:

$$\frac{6}{4} = \frac{30}{x}$$

STEP 1: Cross multiply to get the product of the means and the extremes.

$$\frac{6}{4} \diagup\!\!\!\!\!\diagdown \frac{30}{x}$$

$6 \times x = 6x$, and $4 \times 30 = 120$, so $6x = 120$.

STEP 2: Divide both sides of proportion by the number in front of the *x*, 6.

$$\frac{6x}{6} = \frac{120}{6}$$
$$x = 20$$

To check for accuracy, insert the value of *x* into the proportion and cross multiply.

$$\frac{6}{4} = \frac{30}{\mathbf{20}}$$

$6 \times 20 = 120$, and $4 \times 30 = 120$.

The value obtained for *x* when solving the problem is correct.

Practice 3

Solve for *x* in the following problems.

1. $2:3 :: 8:x$

2. $5:10 :: x:90$

3. $\dfrac{1}{2} = \dfrac{7}{x}$

CALCULATING THE PERCENTAGE STRENGTH IN IV SOLUTIONS

Intravenous solutions are ordered in percentage strengths. The *percentage in a solution* means the number of grams of solute per 100 mL of diluent. These values can be written as a ratio-proportion and used to set up an equation to determine drug amounts in different volumes. A ratio-proportion may be written as a "means to extremes" *equation format*, using colon and equal signs, or in a *fraction format*.

For example, dextrose 5% and water (D_5W) has 5 g of dextrose per 100 mL. To determine how many grams of dextrose are found in 500 mL, set up a ratio and proportion equation using the (1) means : extremes format or (2) fraction format.

(1) extremes : means = means : extremes

$$\text{number of g/100 mL} \rightarrow 5:100 = x:500 \leftarrow \text{unknown number of g/1,000 mL}$$

$$\text{multiply the extremes} \rightarrow 5 \times 500 = 100 \times x \leftarrow \text{multiply the means}$$

$$2{,}500 = 100x$$

$$\text{divide by 100} \rightarrow \frac{2{,}500}{100} = \frac{100x}{100} \leftarrow \text{divide by 100}$$

$$25 \text{ g} = x$$

There are 25 g of dextrose per 500 mL of solution.

(2) fraction format

$$\frac{5}{100} \times \frac{x}{500}$$

Cross multiply.

$$\frac{5}{100} \diagdown\!\!\!\!\diagup^{\times} \frac{x}{500}$$

$$100x = 2{,}500$$

Divide both sides by 100.

$$\frac{100x}{100} = \frac{2{,}500}{100}$$

$$x = 25 \text{ g}$$

There are 25 g of dextrose per 500 mL of solution.

In another example, dextrose 10% and water has 10 g dextrose per 100 mL. To determine how many grams of dextrose are found in 500 mL, again set up a ratio and proportion equation.

(1) Using the means : extremes format:

$$\text{number of g/100 mL} \rightarrow 10 : 100 = x : 500 \leftarrow \text{unknown number of g/500 mL}$$
$$\text{multiply the extremes} \rightarrow 10 \times 500 = 100 \times x \leftarrow \text{multiply the means}$$
$$5{,}000 = 100x$$
$$\text{divide by 100} \rightarrow \frac{5{,}000}{100} = \frac{100x}{100} \leftarrow \text{divide by 100}$$
$$50 \text{ g} = x$$

There are 50 g of dextrose per 500 mL of solution.

(2) Using the fraction format:

$$\frac{10}{100} \times \frac{x}{500}$$

Cross multiply.

$$\frac{10}{100} \times \frac{x}{500}$$
$$100x = 5{,}000$$

Divide both sides by 100.

$$\frac{100x}{100} = \frac{5{,}000}{100}$$
$$x = 50 \text{ g}$$

There are 50 g of dextrose per 500 mL of solution.

Practice 4

Using your method of choice, determine how many grams of drug are found in each solution.

1. How many grams of dextrose are found in 1,000 mL of a 5% solution?

2. How many grams of sodium are found in 1,000 mL of a 3% solution?

3. How many grams of sodium are found in 1,000 mL of a 0.9% solution?

4. How many grams of dextrose are found in 500 mL of a 2.5% solution?

ANSWERS AND EXPLANATIONS TO PRACTICE EXERCISES

Practice 1

1. $\frac{3}{7}$

To convert the ratio 3:7 to a fraction, no calculations are necessary. Simply change the way the numbers are presented.

2. 11:12

To convert the fraction $\frac{11}{12}$ to a ratio, no calculations are necessary. Simply change the way the numbers are presented.

3. 67:100

To convert the decimal 0.67 to a ratio:

STEP 1: Write the decimal as a fraction:
$0.67 = \frac{67}{100}$.

STEP 2: Reduce the fraction to lowest terms, if possible. (This fraction cannot be further reduced.)

STEP 3: State the fraction as a ratio:
$\frac{67}{100} = 67:100$.

4. 1.5

To convert the ratio 3:2 into a decimal:

STEP 1: Write the ratio as a fraction:
3:2 becomes $\frac{3}{2}$.

STEP 2: Convert the fraction to a decimal by dividing the numerator by the denominator: $3 \div 2 = 1.5$.

Therefore, $3:2 = \frac{3}{2} = 1.5$.

5. 22%

To convert the ratio 2:9 to a percent:

STEP 1: Convert the ratio into a decimal.
$2:9 = 2 \div 9 = 0.222\ldots$

STEP 2: Multiply 0.222 by 100 and add the percent symbol. As instructed, round to the nearest percent.
$0.222 \times 100 = 22\%$

6. 4:1

To convert 400% to a ratio:

STEP 1: Write the percent as a fraction:
$400\% = \frac{400}{100}$.

STEP 2: Reduce the fraction to its lowest terms:
$\frac{400}{100} = \frac{4}{1}$.

STEP 3: State the fraction as a ratio: $\frac{4}{1} = 4:1$.

Practice 2

1. 8:9 :: 16:18

To write the fraction proportion $\frac{8}{9} = \frac{16}{18}$ as a ratio-proportion:

STEP 1: Convert each fraction to a ratio.

Thus, $\frac{3}{2}$ becomes 8:9, and $\frac{16}{18}$ becomes 16:18, so 8:9 = 16:18.

STEP 2: Replace the equal sign with a double colon (::).
8:9 :: 16:18

2. $\frac{50}{75} = \frac{100}{150}$

To write the ratio-proportion 50:75 :: 100:150 as a fraction proportion:

STEP 1: Replace the double colon (::) with an equal sign (=): 50:75 = 100:150.

STEP 2: Convert both ratios to fractions:
$\frac{50}{75} = \frac{100}{150}$.

3. No.

To determine if an equation is true and equal, multiply the means and then multiply the extremes.

Means: $7 \times 12 = 84$
Extremes: $6 \times 15 = 90$

If the products are not the same, the equation is not true and equal.

4. Yes.

To determine if an equation is true and equal, multiply the means and then multiply the extremes.

Means: $4 \times 21 = 84$
Extremes: $7 \times 12 = 84$

If the products are the same, the equation is true and equal.

Practice 3

1. 12

$2:3::8:x$

STEP 1: Multiply the means and the extremes.

$3 \times 8 = 24$ (means)
$2 \times x = 2x$ (extremes)

Therefore, $2x = 24$.

STEP 2: Divide both sides of the equation by the number in front of the x, 2.

$2x \div 2 = x$
$24 \div 2 = 12$

Therefore, $x = 12$.

2. 45

$5:10::x:90$

STEP 1: Multiply the means and the extremes.

$10 \times x = 10x$ (means)
$5 \times 90 = 450$ (extremes)

Therefore, $10x = 450$.

STEP 2: Divide both sides of the equation by the number in front of the x, 10.

$10x \div 10 = 1$
$450 \div 10 = 45$

Therefore, $x = 45$.

3. 14

$$\frac{1}{2} = \frac{7}{x}$$

STEP 1: Cross multiply to get the product of the means and the extremes.

$$\frac{1}{2} \diagup\!\!\!\!\diagup \frac{7}{x}$$

$1 \times x = 1x$, and $2 \times 7 = 14$, so $1x = 14$.

STEP 2: Divide both sides of proportion by the number in front of the x, 1.

$$\frac{1x}{1} = \frac{14}{1}$$
$$x = 14$$

Practice 4

1. 50 g

Use the means : extremes method:

$5:100 = x:1,000$ Set up a ratio-proportion equation.

$100x = 5,000$ Multiply the means and extremes.

$x = 50$ Divide both sides by 100 to get x.

$x = 50$ g of dextrose.

Or set up a fraction equation:

$$\frac{5}{100} \times \frac{x}{1,000}$$

Cross multiply.

$$\frac{5}{100} \diagup\!\!\!\!\diagup \frac{x}{1,000}$$
$$100x = 5,000$$

Divide both sides by 100.

$$\frac{100x}{100} = \frac{5,000}{100}$$
$$x = 50 \text{ g}$$

There are 50 g of dextrose per 1,000 mL.

2. 30 g

Use the means : extremes method:

$3 : 100 = x : 1{,}000$ Set up a ratio-proportion equation.

$100x = 3{,}000$ Multiply the means and extremes

$x = 30$ Divide both sides by 100 to get x.

$x = 30$ g of sodium.

Or set up a fraction equation:

$$\frac{3}{100} \times \frac{x}{1{,}000}$$

Cross multiply.

$$\frac{3}{100} \bowtie \frac{x}{1{,}000}$$

$$100x = 3{,}000$$

Divide both sides by 100.

$$\frac{100x}{100} = \frac{3{,}000}{100}$$

$$x = 30 \text{ g}$$

There are 30 g of sodium per 1,000 mL.

3. 9 g

Use the means : extremes method:

$0.9 : 100 = x : 1{,}000$ Set up a ratio-proportion equation.

$100x = 900$ Multiply the means and extremes.

$x = 9$ Divide both sides by 100 to get x.

$x = 9$ g of sodium.

Or set up a fraction equation:

$$\frac{0.9}{100} \times \frac{x}{1{,}000}$$

Cross multiply.

$$\frac{0.9}{100} \bowtie \frac{x}{1{,}000}$$

$$100x = 900$$

Divide both sides by 100.

$$\frac{100x}{100} = \frac{900}{100}$$

$$x = 9 \text{ g}$$

There are 9 g of sodium per 1,000 mL.

4. 12.5 g

Use the means : extremes method:

$2.5 : 100 = x : 500$ Set up a ratio-proportion equation.

$100x = 1{,}250$ Multiply the means and extremes.

$x = 12.5$ Divide both sides by 100 to get x.

There are 12.5 g of dextrose per 500 mL.

Or set up a fraction equation:

$$\frac{2.5}{100} \times \frac{x}{500}$$

Cross multiply.

$$\frac{2.5}{100} \bowtie \frac{x}{500}$$

$$100x = 1{,}250$$

Divide both sides by 100.

$$\frac{100x}{100} = \frac{1{,}250}{100}$$

$$x = 12.5 \text{ g}$$

There are 12.5 g of dextrose per 500 mL.

CHAPTER QUIZ

Solve each problem, then select the correct answer.

1. Convert $1:12::6:72$ to a fraction proportion.

    (A) $\dfrac{1}{12} = \dfrac{6}{72}$ (C) $\dfrac{1}{72} = \dfrac{6}{12}$

    (B) $\dfrac{6}{1} = \dfrac{12}{72}$ (D) $\dfrac{6}{72} = \dfrac{6}{12}$

2. Convert $\dfrac{4}{17} = \dfrac{8}{34}$ to a ratio-proportion.

    (A) $4:8::17:34$ (C) $4:17::8:34$

    (B) $8:4::17:34$ (D) $8:17::4:34$

3. Which numbers represent the *means* in the proportion $9:10::27:30$?

    (A) 9 and 10   (C) 10 and 27

    (B) 9 and 27   (D) 10 and 30

4. Which numbers represent the *extremes* in the proportion $\dfrac{150}{50} = \dfrac{30}{1}$?

    (A) 150 and 30   (C) 50 and 30

    (B) 150 and 1   (D) 50 and 1

5. How many grams of sodium are found in 500 mL of a 3% solution?

    (A) 30 g   (C) 1.5 g

    (B) 15 g   (D) 3 g

6. How many grams of dextrose are found in 250 mL of a 5% solution?

    (A) 1.25 g   (C) 12.5 g

    (B) 0.125 g   (D) 125 g

Solve for x in questions 7–10.

7. $\dfrac{3}{6} = \dfrac{x}{24}$

   (A) 12   (C) 36

   (B) 18   (D) 72

8. $\dfrac{146}{200} = \dfrac{73}{x}$

   (A) 10   (C) 100

   (B) 50   (D) 300

9. $75 : x :: 15 : 1$

   (A) 5   (C) 35

   (B) 15   (D) 75

10. $327 : x :: 109 : 42$

   (A) 109   (C) 654

   (B) 126   (D) 13,644

ANSWERS AND EXPLANATIONS

1.   A

To convert $1:12::6:72$ to a fraction proportion, no calculations are necessary. Simply change the way the numbers are presented.

2.   C

To convert $\frac{4}{17} = \frac{8}{34}$ to a ratio-proportion, no calculations are necessary. Simply change the way the numbers are presented.

3.   C

The numbers in the middle of the equation are referred to as the *means*. In the proportion $9:10::27:30$, the 10 and the 27 are in the middle.

4.   B

Begin by changing the fraction proportion into a ratio proportion. $\frac{150}{50} = \frac{30}{1}$ becomes $150:50::30:1$. The numbers on the outside, or on the ends, of the equations are called the *extremes*. In this proportion, the 150 and the 1 are on the ends.

5.   B

Use the means:extremes method:

$3:100 = x:500$	Set up a ratio-proportion equation.
$100x = 1,500$	Multiply the means and extremes.
$x = 15$	Divide both sides of the equal sign by 100 to get x.

There are 15 g of sodium in 500 mL of solution.

Or set up a fraction equation:

$$\frac{3}{100} \times \frac{x}{500}$$

Cross multiply.

$$\frac{3}{100} \diagup\!\!\!\!\diagdown \frac{x}{500}$$

$$100x = 1,500$$

Divide both sides by 100.

$$\frac{100x}{100} = \frac{1,500}{100}$$

$$x = 15 \text{ g}$$

There are 15 g of sodium per 500 mL of solution.

6.   C

Use the means:extremes method:

$5:100 = x:250$	Set up a ratio-proportion equation.
$100x = 1,250$	Multiply the means and extremes.
$x = 12.5$	Divide both sides by 100 to get x.

There are 12.5 g of dextrose in 250 mL of solution.

Or set up a fraction equation:

$$\frac{5}{100} \times \frac{x}{250}$$

Cross multiply.

$$\frac{5}{100} \diagup\!\!\!\!\diagdown \frac{x}{250}$$

$$100x = 1,250$$

Divide both sides by 100.

$$\frac{100x}{100} = \frac{1,250}{100}$$

$$x = 12.5 \text{ g}$$

There are 12.5 g of dextrose per 250 mL of solution.

7. A

$$\frac{3}{6} = \frac{x}{24}$$

STEP 1: Multiply the means and the extremes.

$6 \times x = 6x$ (means)

$3 \times 24 = 72$ (extremes)

Therefore, $6x = 72$.

STEP 2: Divide both sides of the equation by the number in front of the x, 6.

$6x = 72$

$x = 72 \div 6$

Therefore, $x = 12$.

8. C

$$\frac{146}{200} = \frac{73}{x}$$

STEP 1: Multiply the means and the extremes.

$200 \times 73 = 14{,}600$ (means)

$146 \times x = 146x$ (extremes)

Therefore, $14{,}600 = 146x$.

STEP 2: Divide both sides of the equation by the number in front of the x, 146.

$14{,}600 = 146x$

$14{,}600 \div 146 = x$

Therefore, $x = 100$.

9. A

$75 : x :: 15 : 1$

STEP 1: Multiply the means and the extremes.

$x \times 15 = 15x$ (means)

$75 \times 1 = 75$ (extremes)

Therefore, $15x = 75$.

STEP 2: Divide both sides of the equation by the number in front of the x, 15.

$15x = 75$

$x = 75 \div 15$

Therefore, $x = 5$.

10. B

$327 : x :: 109 : 42$

STEP 1: Multiply the means and the extremes.

$x \times 109 = 109x$ (means)

$327 \times 42 = 13{,}734$ (extremes)

Therefore, $109x = 13{,}734$.

STEP 2: Divide both sides of the equation by the number in front of the x, 109.

$109x = 13{,}734$

$x = 13{,}734 \div 109$

Therefore, $x = 126$.

CHAPTER 6

Rates

A rate is a ratio that compares two different kinds of numbers, such as miles per hour when traveling or price per gallon when filling the tank with gas. Rates are used in many everyday tasks, such as grocery shopping and traveling, as well as in calculating medications and IV fluids.

Miles per hour and feet per second are both rates of speed. The number of dollars you make per hour is your rate of pay. The words *per* and *for* indicate that you are dealing with a rate. For example, suppose 4 oranges are selling for $1.00. This means that oranges are selling at a rate of $1.00 per 4 oranges. To determine the price per orange, the total cost of $1.00 is divided by the number of items, 4. Therefore, the price per orange is:

$$\frac{\$1.00}{4} = \$0.25, \text{ or 25 cents.}$$

This chapter will cover solving rate problems using proportions. It will also introduce the use of formulas when solving problems. Chapter 8: Basic Problem Solving and Strategies for Dosage Calculation will cover these topics in more depth. Using rates to calculate IV fluids and medications will be covered in Chapter 11.

UNDERSTANDING RATES

Since a rate can be expressed as both a ratio and a fraction, problems involving rates can be solved using proportions. Many problems involving rates, including medication orders, are word problems. To solve these types of problems using ratios and proportions, the first step is to translate them into an equation.

Everyday Rate Problems

Say, for example, that Joan needs to purchase a sheet of 20 stamps at the post office. Each stamp costs 49 cents. Practice building an equation to determine how much the entire roll of stamps will cost.

Set up the equation based on the information provided.

STEP 1: One stamp costs 49 cents.

Write this as $1:49$ or $\frac{1}{49}$.

STEP 2: There are 20 stamps in a sheet, but the cost of the sheet is not known.

Write this as $20:x$ or $\frac{20}{x}$.

STEP 3: Write the ratios as a proportion.

$1:49 :: 20:x$, or $\frac{1}{49} = \frac{20}{x}$.

STEP 4: Solve for x. (If you need to review this process, go back to Chapter 5: Ratios and Proportions.)

$1x = 980$

$x = 980$

This means that 20 stamps will cost 980 cents, or $9.80 per sheet.

Chances are, most people would be able to calculate the cost of a sheet of stamps without actually setting up the problem as an equation. This is just an example of how we use rates in our everyday lives.

Here's another example. The 5-pound family pack of ground beef is on sale for $11.95 at the local market. How much does the ground beef cost per pound?

Set up the equation based on the information provided.

STEP 1: The 5-pound package of ground beef costs $11.95.

Write this as $5:11.95$ or $\frac{5}{11.95}$.

STEP 2: You want to know how much 1 pound of the ground beef costs.

Write this as $1:x$ or $\frac{1}{x}$.

STEP 3: Write the ratios as a proportion.

$5:11.95 :: 1:x$, or $\frac{5}{11.95} = \frac{1}{x}$.

STEP 4: Solve for x. (If you need to review this process, go back to Chapter 5.)

$5x = 11.95$

$x = 2.39$

This means that ground beef in the 5-pound family pack costs $2.39 per pound.

When setting up a rate problem, make sure that you are clear on what you are trying to determine. For example, if the left side of the equation is set up in cost per pound, the right side must also be in cost per pound. If the numbers are reversed on the right side and are stated in pounds per cost, the answer will be incorrect. It is fairly easy to spot this error, as the answer will not be logical. In the previous example, if the right side of the equation were set up incorrectly, the answer would have been 41.8 cents per pound, which doesn't make sense because 41.8 cents times 5 is only $2.09.

Practice 1

1. If gas costs $2.59 per gallon, how much will it cost to put 12 gallons of gas in the car?

2. Dan drove 1,575 miles in 22.5 hours while on vacation. How many miles was he driving per hour?

3. Grapes are on sale for $1.29 per pound. How much will 3.5 pounds of grapes cost, rounded to the nearest cent?

4. Bill is using a water sprinkler on his lawn that delivers 5 gallons of water per minute. How many gallons of water will he use if he leaves the sprinkler running for 20 minutes?

5. A day care center serves each child 4 ounces of juice each morning. How many ounces of juice will the center need each day to serve 55 children?

More Everyday Rate Problems

Many everyday problems involve rates of speed, using distance and time.

For example, say it is 81.25 miles from John's house to the airport. Assuming that he drives at 65 miles per hour the entire distance, how long will it take him to drive to the airport?

Set up the equation based on the information provided.

STEP 1: John is driving 65 miles per hour.

Write this as $65:1$ or $\frac{65}{1}$.

STEP 2: You want to know how long it will take to drive 81.25 miles.

Write this as $81.25:x$ or $\frac{81.25}{x}$.

STEP 3: Write the ratios as a proportion.

$65:1 :: 81.25:x$, or $\frac{65}{1} = \frac{81.25}{x}$.

STEP 4: Solve for x. (If you need to review this process, go back to Chapter 5.)

$65x = 81.25$

$x = 1.25$

It will take 1.25 hours, or 1 hour and 15 minutes, to drive to the airport.

This problem can also be solved using a handy formula. This formula comes directly from the proportion calculation, but one multiplication step has already been done for you. Therefore, learning the formula gives you a shortcut.

Depending on what you already know and what you need to find out, there are three versions of this formula.

1. Rate equals distance divided by time: $r = \frac{d}{t}$.

2. Distance equals rate times time: $d = r \times t$.

3. Time equals distance divided by rate: $t = \frac{d}{r}$.

In the example above, you know that it is 81.25 miles from John's house to the airport. Assuming that he drives 65 miles an hour the entire distance, how long will it take him to drive to the airport?

In this example, you are solving for, or determining, the amount of *time* it will take to make the trip. You are given the *distance* (81.25 miles) and the rate or *speed* of travel (65mph).

$t = 81.25 \div 65$

$t = 1.25$

The time it takes John to drive from his house to the airport is, therefore, 1.25 hours.

In another example, let's say you rode your bike 3 hours and traveled 15 miles. What was your rate of speed? Use the rate formula: $r = \frac{d}{t}$.

r = 15 miles ÷ 3 hours

r = 5 miles per hour

Now let's say you rode your bike at a rate of 8 miles per hour for four hours. How many miles did you travel? This time, use the distance formula: $d = r \times t$.

d = 8 miles per hour × 4 hours

d = 32 miles

> **Math Tip:** For most people, one method of calculating a rate comes more easily than other methods. Use whichever method you are more comfortable with to solve the practice problems.

> **Math Tip:** Using a formula to set up a rate question makes solving the problem quick and easy. The three basic formulas for calculating distance, time, and speed rate are:
>
> 1. Rate equals distance divided by time ($r = \frac{d}{t}$).
> 2. Distance equals rate times time ($d = r \times t$).
> 3. Time equals distance divided by rate ($t = \frac{d}{r}$).

Practice 2

Solve the problems using one of the formulas introduced in this chapter.

1. How long will it take to travel 693 miles driving 58.5 miles per hour?

2. How far will you have traveled if you fly at 487 miles per hour for 1.75 hours?

3. How fast do you need to drive to make a 350-mile trip in seven hours?

4. John travels 560 miles per day. How many miles will he travel in five days?

5. A mouse travels 150 feet a minute. How long will it take the mouse to run 3,750 feet if it runs without stopping?

ANSWERS AND EXPLANATIONS TO PRACTICE EXERCISES

Practice 1

1. $31.08

Set up the equation based on the information provided.

STEP 1: Gas costs $2.59 per gallon.

Write this as $1:2.59$ or $\frac{1}{2.59}$.

STEP 2: You want to know how much 12 gallons of gas will cost.

Write this as $12:x$ or $\frac{12}{x}$.

STEP 3: Write the ratios as a proportion.

$1:2.59 :: 12:x$, or $\frac{1}{2.59} = \frac{12}{x}$.

STEP 4: Solve for x.

$1x = 31.08$

$x = 31.08$

This means that 12 gallons of gas will cost $31.08.

2. 70 mph

Set up the equation based on the information provided.

STEP 1: Dan drove 1,575 miles in 22.5 hours while on vacation.

Write this as $1,575:22.5$ or $\frac{1,575}{22.5}$.

STEP 2: You want to know how many miles he was driving per hour.

Write this as $x:1$ or $\frac{x}{1}$.

STEP 3: Write the ratios as a proportion.

$1,575:22.5 :: x:1$, or $\frac{1,575}{22.5} = \frac{x}{1}$.

STEP 4: Solve for x.

$22.5x = 1,575$

$x = 70$

Dan was driving at 70 miles per hour.

3. $4.52

Set up the equation based on the information provided.

STEP 1: Grapes cost $1.29.

Write this as $1:1.29$ or $\frac{1}{1.29}$.

STEP 2: You want to know how much 3.5 pounds of grapes will cost.

Write this as $3.5:x$ or $\frac{3.5}{x}$.

STEP 3: Write the ratios as a proportion.

$1:1.29 :: 3.5:x$, or $\frac{1}{1.29} = \frac{3.5}{x}$.

STEP 4: Solve for x and round to the nearest cent.

$1x = 4.515$

$x = 4.52$

This means that 3.5 pounds of grapes will cost $4.52.

4. 100 gallons of water

Set up the equation based on the information provided.

STEP 1: The sprinkler delivers five gallons of water per minute.

Write this as $5:1$ or $\frac{5}{1}$.

STEP 2: You want to know how much water will be used in 20 minutes.

Write this as $x:20$ or $\frac{x}{20}$.

STEP 3: Write the ratios as a proportion.

$5:1 :: x:20$, or $\frac{5}{1} = \frac{x}{20}$.

STEP 4: Solve for x.

$1x = 100$

$x = 100$

The sprinkler will use 100 gallons of water over 20 minutes.

5. 220 ounces of juice

Set up the equation based on the information provided.

STEP 1: The day care serves 4 ounces of juice to each child.

Write this as 4:1 or $\frac{4}{1}$.

STEP 2: You want to know how much juice is needed to serve 55 children.

Write this as x:55 or $\frac{x}{55}$.

STEP 3: Write the ratios as a proportion.

$4:1 :: x:55$ or $\frac{4}{1} = \frac{x}{55}$.

STEP 4: Solve for x.

$1x = 220$

$x = 220$

So 220 ounces of juice will be required to serve each of the children 4 ounces.

Practice 2

1. 11.8 hours or 11 hours and 48 minutes

Time equals distance divided by rate: $t = \frac{d}{r}$.

$t = 693 \div 58.5$

2. 852.25 miles

Distance equals rate times time: $d = r \times t$.

$d = 487 \times 1.75$

3. 50 miles per hour

Rate equals distance divided by time: $r = \frac{d}{t}$.

$r = 350 \div 7$

4. 2,800 miles

$d = r \times t$

$d = 560 \times 5$

5. 25 minutes

$t = \frac{d}{r}$

$t = 3,750 \div 150$

CHAPTER QUIZ

1. Eggs cost $2.76 per dozen. What is the cost per egg?

   (A) 21 cents   (C) 23 cents

   (B) 22 cents   (D) 24 cents

2. John earns $8.75 per hour. How much will he earn in an 80-hour pay period?

   (A) $700   (C) $1,125

   (B) $1,095   (D) $1,300

3. Your soup recipe requires 12 ounces of water for two servings. How many ounces of water are needed if you wish to make six servings of soup?

   (A) 24 ounces   (C) 48 ounces

   (B) 36 ounces   (D) 72 ounces

4. Athletic socks are sold in packages of three for $10.95. How much does each pair of socks cost?

   (A) $1.62   (C) $3.65

   (B) $2.99   (D) $3.95

5. There are 22 students in Mrs. Smith's first grade class. If she brings cookies for the entire class, how many cookies will be needed if each child eats two cookies?

   (A) 22   (C) 66

   (B) 44   (D) 88

6. It is 299 miles from St. Louis to Chicago. If it takes 45 minutes to make the trip by airplane, how fast is the plane flying?

   (A) 6.64 miles per hour

   (B) 66.4 miles per hour

   (C) 66.4 miles per minute

   (D) 6.64 miles per minute

7. It takes Ed one hour to drive 12 miles in rush hour traffic on the interstate. How many miles per hour is Ed driving?

   (A) 5 mph

   (B) 12 mph

   (C) 16 mph

   (D) 24 mph

8. If a train is traveling at 82 miles per hour, how far can it travel in 13 hours and 15 minutes?

   (A) 1,065.7 miles

   (B) 1,078.3 miles

   (C) 1,086.5 miles

   (D) 1,097.1 miles

9. The speed limit on the interstate is 70 miles per hour. How many miles can you travel in $7\frac{1}{2}$ hours if you drive the entire time at the speed limit?

   (A) 495 miles

   (B) 511 miles

   (C) 515 miles

   (D) 525 miles

10. Sue is traveling across the country on vacation. How many miles per hour will she need to drive if she wishes to travel 500 miles per day and drives 8 hours each day?

   (A) 40 mph

   (B) 56.8 mph

   (C) 62.5 mph

   (D) 65.1 mph

ANSWERS AND EXPLANATIONS

1. C

STEP 1: Eggs cost $2.76 per dozen.

Write this as $2.76 : 12$ or $\frac{2.76}{12}$.

STEP 2: You want to know how much one egg costs.

Write this as $x : 1$ or $\frac{x}{1}$.

STEP 3: Write the ratios as a proportion.

$2.76 : 12 :: x : 1$, or $\frac{2.76}{12} = \frac{x}{1}$.

STEP 4: Solve for x.

$2.76 = 12x$ (Divide each side of the equation by 12.)

$0.23 = x$

2. A

STEP 1: John earns $8.75 per hour.

Write this as $8.75 : 1$ or $\frac{8.75}{1}$.

STEP 2: He works 80 hours in a pay period.

Write this as $x : 80$ or $\frac{x}{80}$.

STEP 3: Write the ratios as a proportion.

$8.75 : 1 :: x : 80$, or $\frac{8.75}{1} = \frac{x}{80}$.

STEP 4: Solve for x.

$1x = 700$

$x = 700$

3. B

STEP 1: Your soup recipe requires 12 ounces of water for two servings.

Write this as $12 : 2$ or $\frac{12}{2}$.

STEP 2: How many ounces of water are needed to make six servings of soup?

Write this as $x : 6$ or $\frac{x}{6}$.

STEP 3: Write the ratios as a proportion.

$12 : 2 :: x : 6$, or $\frac{12}{2} = \frac{x}{6}$.

STEP 4: Solve for x.

$2x = 72$ (Divide both sides of the equation by 2.)

$x = 36$

4. C

STEP 1: Athletic socks are sold in packages of three for $10.95.

Write this as $3 : 10.95$ or $\frac{3}{10.95}$.

STEP 2: How much does one pair of socks cost?

Write this as $1 : x$ or $\frac{1}{x}$.

STEP 3: Write the ratios as a proportion.

$3 : 10.95 :: 1 : x$, or $\frac{3}{10.95} = \frac{1}{x}$.

STEP 4: Solve for x.

$3x = 10.95$ (Divide both sides of the equation by 3.)

$x = 3.65$

5. B

STEP 1: There are 22 students in class.

Write this as $1 : 22$ or $\frac{1}{22}$.

STEP 2: How many cookies will be needed if each child eats two cookies?

Write this as $2 : x$ or $\frac{2}{x}$.

STEP 3: Write the ratios as a proportion.

$1 : 22 :: 2 : x$, or $\frac{1}{22} = \frac{2}{x}$.

STEP 4: Solve for x.

$1x = 44$

$x = 44$

6. D

Rate equals distance divided by time. In this problem, your answer will be in miles per minute.

$$r = \frac{d}{t}$$
$$r = \frac{299}{45}$$
$$r = 6.64$$

7. B

Rate equals distance divided by time.

$$r = \frac{d}{t}$$
$$r = \frac{12}{1}$$
$$r = 12$$

8. C

Distance equals rate times time. In this problem, you need to remember that 13 hours and 15 minutes is equal to 13.25 hours.

$$d = r \times t$$
$$d = 82 \times 13.25$$
$$d = 1,086.5$$

9. D

Distance equals rate times time. Remember that $7\frac{1}{2}$ hours is the same as 7.5 hours.

$$d = r \times t$$
$$d = 70 \times 7.5$$
$$d = 525$$

10. C

Rate equals distance divided by time.

$$r = \frac{d}{t}$$
$$r = \frac{500}{8}$$
$$r = 62.5$$

② Applications

CHAPTER 7

Systems of Measurement

Nurses use a variety of measurement systems on a daily basis. It is important to understand the various systems and to be able to convert between them. While the metric system is the system most commonly used in health care, the apothecary system may still be seen, and many patients rely on the household system of measurement when taking medications in their homes.

This chapter will present all three systems and cover methods of converting between the systems. An easy to use "Conversion at a Glance" table is included to facilitate the conversion process. This chapter will also address drugs measured in units, milliequivalents, percentages, ratios, and inches as well as temperature conversions and military time.

THE APOTHECARY SYSTEM

The apothecary system is one of the oldest systems of measurement used when calculating drug dosages. While the metric system is now the standard system of measurement for drug dosages, some physicians still use the apothecary system when prescribing certain medications such as aspirin.

The basic unit of measurement used for weight in the apothecary system is the grain (gr). The weight of a grain is based on the weight of a single grain of wheat. The three units used for measuring volume in the apothecary system are the minim (m), dram (dr or ℨ), and ounce (oz or ℥). The symbols for drams and ounces are easily confused for the number 3 and should never be used.

Apothecary measurements are considered to be approximate measurements, so they are used less frequently when working with medications. For example, a grain is equivalent to 60–65 mg—conversions between the metric and apothecary system are not precise. Whenever possible, it is preferable to convert an apothecary measurement to a metric measurement.

The apothecary ounce has become an accepted component of the household measurement system, which is covered later in this chapter.

HOUSEHOLD MEASUREMENTS

Household measurements are calculated using measuring devices commonly used for cooking such as measuring cups and measuring spoons. The household measurement system is the least accurate of all three systems due to variances in household measuring devices. For example, a household teaspoon can hold anywhere from 4 to 7 mL of fluid.

The measuring cup is the most common measuring device found in the home. Most measuring cups are calibrated in ounces as well as in $\frac{1}{4}$-cup increments. It is important to note that some units of liquid measurement used in the household system, such as pints and quarts, are also used in the apothecary system. Arabic numbers such as 1 teaspoon or $2\frac{1}{4}$ cups are used to express quantities in the household system.

Many households also have a 1-ounce measuring device that is calibrated in teaspoons, tablespoons, and milliliters. Some drug manufacturers package a 1-ounce measuring device with their product to assist in measuring correct drug dosages. This 1-ounce measuring device is very similar to the medicine cups used to measure liquid medications in the health care setting.

The smallest unit of measurement used in the household system is the drop; however, drops can vary significantly in size and are generally considered an inaccurate form of measurement for most medications. The exception to this is when a dropper provided by the drug manufacturer and packaged with the medication is used to measure the dosage. Eye drops and ear drops are examples of medications administered using a dropper.

While some providers still dose oral suspensions in teaspoons, tablespoons, or ounces, best practice is to always dose in milliliters. Regardless of which unit is used in a medication prescription, patients should never be expected to perform any conversions or calculations. It is important that the patient have the proper measuring device for the prescription. To help prevent errors in dosing, pediatric medications are frequently packaged with a dropper or a hollow-handle spoon calibrated in teaspoons, tablespoons, and milliliters to assure that parents can accurately measure the smaller dosages commonly associated with children's medications.

The Most Common Household Units of Measurement with Equivalent Liquid Volumes

Household Unit	Liquid Volume
60 drops	1 teaspoon
3 teaspoons	1 tablespoon
2 tablespoons	1 ounce
8 ounces	1 cup
2 cups	1 pint
2 pints	1 quart
4 quarts	1 gallon

Sometimes a medication label gives instructions in a unit of household measurement that the nurse does not have available.

For example, the label instructions may tell the nurse to administer 2 tablespoons of medication, but the nurse only has a measuring device marked in teaspoons. Knowing that there are 3 teaspoons in one tablespoon, the nurse can easily complete this conversion by solving for x.

$$\frac{3}{1} = \frac{x}{2}$$

Cross multiply to find the answer: $3 \times 2 = 1x$.

$x = 6$, so the nurse would administer 6 teaspoons of medication.

> **Math Tip:** If you need to review the steps required to solve for x, go back and review Chapters 5 and 6.

Practice 1

Complete the following household conversions.

1. How many tablespoons are in 3 ounces?

2. How many ounces are in half a cup?

THE METRIC SYSTEM

Most parts of the world use the metric system of measurement. It is also the system most commonly used to measure medications. The metric system is based on the decimal system, which means that it eliminates most fractions and simplifies most dosage calculations.

The three basic units of measurement in the metric system are:

1. **Gram (g).** Used to measure weight.
2. **Liter (L).** Used to measure volume (usually liquids).
3. **Meter (m).** Used to measure length.

While grams and liters are used in dosage calculations, meters are usually used for measuring height or size.

> **Math Tip:** A capital *L* is the currently preferred abbreviation for liter. A lowercase *l* can be mistaken for the number 1 (one), possibly resulting in a medication error.

> **Math Tip:** The abbreviation *cc* stands for cubic centimeter, which has the same volume as a milliliter (mL). While they have historically been used interchangeably, when handwritten, *cc* may be misread as *u*, which represents units. The current recommendation is to use *mL* rather than *cc*.

The metric system uses common prefixes to indicate the numeric value of the unit being considered. The most commonly used are listed in the table below.

Prefix	Abbreviation	Numeric Value	Meaning
Kilo	k	1,000	one thousand times
Centi	c	0.01 or $\frac{1}{100}$	one hundredth
Milli	m	0.001 or $\frac{1}{1,000}$	one thousandth
Micro	mc	0.000001 or $\frac{1}{1,000,000}$	one millionth

The prefix is added to the unit of measurement to describe the size amount of the measurement. For example, a kilogram is equal to 1,000 g, and a centimeter is equal to $\frac{1}{100}$ of a meter. Converting within the metric system is the same as converting within the household system.

In the metric system, the abbreviation for the unit of measure always follows the number representing the quantity, such as 10 mL. Decimals are used, rather than fractions, when the number is less than a whole. For example, 1.5 mL would be used rather than $1\frac{1}{2}$ mL. Remember to eliminate trailing zeros by writing 5 mL rather than 5.0 mL, which could be misread as 50 mL. For numbers that are less than 1, always use a zero in front of the decimal point. For example, write 0.75 mL rather than .75 mL, which could be misread as 75 mL.

> **Math Tip:** It is important to have a good understanding of decimals before attempting to calculate drug dosages using the metric system. Chapter 3 provides a good review of working with decimals.

For example, the physician has ordered 1.5 g cefazolin sodium, but you want to know how many milligrams that is. If you know that there are 1,000 mg in 1 g, you can easily set up this problem and solve for x.

$$\frac{1,000 \text{ mg}}{1 \text{ g}} = \frac{x \text{ mg}}{1.5 \text{ g}}$$

Cross multiply to find the answer: $1,000 \times 1.5 = 1 \times x$.

Because $1,500 = x$, there are 1,500 mg of cefazolin sodium in 1.5 g.

OTHER SYSTEMS OF MEASUREMENT

The *avoirdupois system* derives from the French term *avoir du pois* meaning "goods of weight," referring to goods sold by weight. This system is based on the household measurement of a pound and is used when purchasing items by weight. It is not currently used in calculating drug dosages but may be referred to in some texts.

Some drugs, such as insulin, heparin, vitamins, and penicillin, are measured by a special designation called a *unit*. Insulin is manufactured in solutions that contain 100 units per milliliter and is labeled U-100. The U-100 indicates the strength, or number, of units per mL. Vitamins may be measured in *international units (IU)* or *United States Pharmacopeia (USP) units*.

Doses of electrolytes, such as potassium, may be measured in *milliequivalents (mEq)*. An equivalent (Eq) is the molecular weight of an ion divided by the number of hydrogen ions it reacts with. A milliequivalent is $\frac{1}{1,000}$ of an equivalent.

Percentages are commonly used to describe the strength of a medication in a solution. Examples include 5% DW, which contains 5% dextrose in water, or a topical cream or ointment like 2.5% triamcinolone, which contains 25 mg of the drug in a 1,000 mg base.

A *ratio* expresses the relationship between two substances in a solution. Epinephrine with a local anesthetic used for subcutaneous injection is supplied in a ratio of 1 : 100,000, or 1 part epinephrine to 100,000 parts solution.

Nitroglycerin ointment is the only commonly prescribed drug that is ordered in *inches*. Specially calibrated paper is provided with the medication by the manufacturer so that the dose can be measured. The ointment is squeezed onto the paper along the measurement line before it is applied to the body.

> **Math Tip:** Chapters 4 and 5 contain information regarding working with percentages and ratios. Reviewing them may be helpful.

Practice 2

1. How many grams are equivalent to 3.5 kilograms?

2. How many milliliters are in 4 liters?

CONVERSION AT A GLANCE

To understand better the relationship and equivalents among the apothecary, household, and metric systems, please refer to the following conversion chart. Although you may never encounter an order written in apothecary units, it is important to recognize apothecary units so that you can prevent medication errors. If you do encounter an order written in drams, grains, or minims, *always contact the provider* and ask them to reorder the medication in a more standard form.

Not all conversions will be precise; some are approximate. You should refer to your facility's policies and procedures for converting between systems.

Apothecary	Household	Metric
Solid (Weight) Measurements		
1 grain (gr)	—	60–65 milligrams (mg)
480 grains (gr)	1 ounce (oz)	28.35 grams (g)
—	2.2 pounds (lb)	1 kilogram (kg)
1 minim (m)	1 drop (gtt)	0.06 milliliter (mL)
15–16 minims (m)	15–16 drops (gtt)	1 milliliter (mL)
Fluid (Liquid) Measurements		
1 dram (dr)	1 teaspoon (tsp)	5 milliliters (mL)
$\frac{1}{2}$ ounce (oz)	1 tablespoon (Tbs)	15 milliliters (mL)
1 ounce (oz)	2 tablespoons (Tbs)	30 milliliters (mL)
8 ounces (oz)	$\frac{1}{2}$ pint (pt) or 1 cup (c)	240 milliliters (mL)
16 ounces (oz)	1 pint (pt) or 2 cups (c)	480 milliliters (mL)
32 ounces (oz)	1 quart (qt), 2 pints (pt), or 4 cups (c)	960 milliliters (mL)
128 ounces (oz)	1 gallon (gal), 4 quarts (qt), 8 pints (pt), or 16 cups (c)	3,840 milliliters (mL)

The equivalents listed in the following box are used on a daily basis when calculating dosages as well as intake and output. Memorize these equivalents, and your dosage calculations will be much easier.

Common Equivalents

30 mL = 1 ounce (oz)

240 mL = 8 ounces (oz) = 1 cup

5 mL = 1 teaspoon (tsp)

15 mL = 1 tablespoon (Tbs) = 3 teaspoons (tsp)

1 kilogram (kg) = 2.2 pounds (lb)

CONVERSION STRATEGIES

It is important that you be able to convert between different systems of measurement with accuracy. Once you have memorized the basic conversions/equivalents, the process is simple. Follow the basic principles you have already learned to make the conversions. Pay close attention to the abbreviations and units of measurement you are working with. For example, mistaking grains (gr) for grams (g) or confusing milliliters (mL) with millimeters (mm) will result in incorrect calculations.

In some cases, you will convert within the same system, as you did when you solved the problems in Practices 1 and 2. Other times, you will convert between systems.

For example, when calculating the patient's intake and output, you note that the patient had the following liquids on his breakfast tray:

- 6 oz coffee
- 4 oz orange juice
- 8 oz milk

Your facility requires that intake and output be documented using milliliters (mL) rather than ounces. How many mL of fluid did your patient consume?

STEP 1: Total the number of ounces consumed.

6 oz + 4 oz + 8 oz = 18 oz

STEP 2: Convert the ounces into mL using the appropriate conversion factor/equivalent.

1 oz = 30 mL

STEP 3: Set up the problem and solve for x to find the answer.

$$\frac{1 \text{ oz}}{30 \text{ mL}} = \frac{18 \text{ oz}}{x \text{ mL}}$$

Cross multiply: $1 \times x = 30 \times 18$.

Therefore, $1x = 540$.

STEP 4: Label the answer correctly. This is a very important step! The problem required you to convert from ounces to milliliters, so the answer is 540 mL.

Converting a patient's weight from pounds (lb) into kilograms (kg) is necessary when a medication is ordered based on a specific number of mg of medication to be given per kg of body weight. This is commonly required when giving medications to pediatric patients (Chapter 12) but is useful in other situations as well.

For example, say Mr. Johnson weighs 160 lb. How many kg does he weigh?

STEP 1: You already know that 2.2 lb = 1 kg. This will be your conversion factor.

STEP 2: Set up the problem.

$$\frac{2.2 \text{ lb}}{1 \text{ kg}} = \frac{160 \text{ lb}}{x \text{ kg}}$$

STEP 3: Cross multiply: $2.2 \times x = 1 \times 160$.

Therefore, $2.2x = 160$. Divide both sides of the equation by 2.2: $x = 72.72$.

STEP 4: Label the answer correctly. Mr. Johnson weighs 72.72 kg.

Practice 3

1. The physician has ordered two tablespoons of aluminum hydroxide, an antacid, for your patient. How many milliliters would you administer?

2. The physician has ordered aspirin gr *x* for your patient. How many milligrams (mg) of aspirin will the patient receive?

TEMPERATURE CONVERSIONS

Converting temperatures from Fahrenheit to Celsius and Celsius to Fahrenheit is sometimes required when administering medications, such as antipyretics, in response to a specific temperature.

To convert Fahrenheit to Celsius, subtract 32 from the temperature in Fahrenheit and divide the difference by 1.8.

$(F - 32) \div 1.8 = $ degrees Celsius

For example: 98.6 °F = _____ °C?

$(98.6 - 32) = 66.6$
$66.6 \div 1.8 = 37$

Therefore, 98.6 °F = 37 °C.

To convert Celsius to Fahrenheit, multiply the temperature in Celsius by 1.8 and add 32.

$(C \times 1.8) + 32 = $ degrees Fahrenheit

For example: 39 °C = _____ °F?

$(39 \times 1.8) = 70.2$
$70.2 + 32 = 102.2$

Therefore, 39 °C = 102.2 °F.

> **Math Tip:** When performing a temperature conversion, round to the nearest tenth. For example, 38.82 would become 38.8, but 38.87 would become 38.9. Refer to Chapter 3 for a review on rounding decimals if necessary.

Practice 4

1. 100 °F = _____ °C

2. 38 °C = _____ °F

MILITARY TIME

Some health care facilities use military time for all medication orders and documentation. This method of time is based on a 24-hour clock. Military time helps prevent medication errors and clarifies documentation, because it eliminates the use of *AM* and *PM*. Some facilities refer to military time as "computer time," since many computer systems use the same method of tracking time.

There may be occasions when you need to convert from traditional time to military time or from military time to traditional time.

Converting from traditional time to military time is very easy if you follow a few simple steps.

STEP 1: When converting an AM time, simply omit the colon and AM designation and add a zero (0) before the time if the hour is between 1 and 9.

2:15 AM becomes 0215.

11:41 AM becomes 1141.
(Note that since the hour was greater than 9, no zero was added.)

When writing numbers between 12:01 AM and 12:59 AM, replace the hour (12) with two zeros (00) in front of the time.

12:15 AM becomes 0015.

12:39 AM becomes 0039.

STEP 2: When converting a PM time, omit the colon and the PM designation and add 1200 to the time.

9:30 PM becomes 930 + 1200 = 2130.

Midnight, or 12:00 AM, becomes 1200 + 1200 = 2400. (Alternatively, midnight can be expressed as 0000 in military time.)

> **Math Tip:** In military time, the time is always expressed using four digits.

Converting from military time to traditional time is just as simple.

STEP 1: When converting to an AM time, omit any zero(s) in front of the number, insert the colon, and add the AM designation.

0617 becomes 6:17 AM.

STEP 2: When converting to a PM time, subtract 1200, insert a colon, and add the PM designation.

1745 becomes 5:45 PM.

Practice 5

Convert the following to military time.

1. 1:55 AM

2. 11:40 PM

Convert the following to traditional time.

3. 0812

4. 2225

ANSWERS AND EXPLANATIONS TO PRACTICE EXERCISES

Practice 1

1. 6 tablespoons

$$\frac{2\,\text{Tbs}}{1\,\text{oz}} = \frac{x\,\text{Tbs}}{3\,\text{oz}}$$

Cross multiply:

$$2 \times 3 = 1 \times x$$
$$6 = 1x$$
$$6 = x$$

2. 4 ounces

Convert $\frac{1}{2}$ to a decimal of 0.5.

$$\frac{8\,\text{oz}}{1\,\text{c}} = \frac{x\,\text{oz}}{0.5\,\text{c}}$$

Cross multiply:

$$8 \times 0.5 = 1 \times x$$
$$4 = 1x$$
$$4 = x$$

Practice 2

1. 3,500 g

$$\frac{1,000\,\text{g}}{1\,\text{kg}} = \frac{x\,\text{g}}{3.5\,\text{kg}}$$

Cross multiply:

$$1,000 \times 3.5 = 1 \times x$$
$$3,500 = 1x$$
$$3,500 = x$$

2. 4,000 mL

$$\frac{1,000\,\text{mL}}{1\,\text{L}} = \frac{x\,\text{mL}}{4\,\text{L}}$$

Cross multiply:

$$1,000 \times 4 = 1 \times x$$
$$4,000 = 1x$$
$$4,000 = x$$

Practice 3

1. 30 mL

$$\frac{1\,\text{Tbs}}{15\,\text{mL}} = \frac{2\,\text{Tbs}}{x\,\text{mL}}$$

Cross multiply:

$$1 \times x = 15 \times 2$$
$$1x = 30$$
$$x = 30$$

Remember to label the answer correctly. In this problem, you were trying to determine the number of mL in 2 tablespoons, so the answer is labeled in milliliters (mL).

2. 600–650 mg

This is a tricky problem, because the conversion between the apothecary system and the metric system is not exact. Your first step will be to convert the Roman numeral into an Arabic numeral: $x = 10$.

$$\frac{1\,\text{gr}}{60\text{–}65\,\text{mg}} = \frac{10\,\text{gr}}{x\,\text{mg}}$$

Cross multiply:

$$1 \times x = 60\text{–}65 \times 10$$
$$1x = 600\text{–}650$$

Remember to label the answer correctly. In this problem, you were trying to determine the number of mg in 10 grains, so the answer is labeled in milligrams (mg).

Practice 4

1. 37.8 °C

  (F – 32) ÷ 1.8 = degrees Celsius
(100 – 32) ÷ 1.8 = degrees Celsius
      68 ÷ 1.8 = 37.77

In this problem, you would round to the nearest tenth, so 37.77 rounds to 37.8. Therefore, 100 °F = 37.8 °C.

2. 100.4 °F

  (C × 1.8) + 32 = degrees Fahrenheit
(38 × 1.8) + 32 = degrees Fahrenheit
      68.4 + 32 = 100.4

Therefore, 38 °C = 100.4 °F.

Practice 5

1. 0155

Delete the colon and AM designation and add a zero (0) in front of the 1.

2. 2340

Delete the colon and PM designation; add 1200.

3. 8:12 AM

Delete the zero, insert the colon, and add the AM designation.

4. 10:25 PM

Subtract 1200, insert the colon, and add the PM designation.

CHAPTER QUIZ

Solve the following problems and select the best answer.

1. How many ounces are in 2 cups?

    (A) 4   (C) 8

    (B) 12   (D) 16

2. How many teaspoons are in a tablespoon?

    (A) 2   (C) 5

    (B) 3   (D) 15

3. How many mL are in one (1) ounce?

    (A) 3   (C) 15

    (B) 10   (D) 30

4. 0.75 g = _____ mg?

    (A) 7.5 mg   (C) 750 mg

    (B) 75 mg   (D) 7,500 mg

5. 195 lb = _____ kg?

    (A) 86.33   (C) 886.30

    (B) 88.63   (D) 868.33

6. The physician has ordered four ounces of citrate of magnesia. How many mL should be given?

   (A) 30   (C) 90
   (B) 45   (D) 120

7. Convert 101.2 °F to Celsius.

   (A) 38.0   (C) 38.4
   (B) 38.2   (D) 38.6

8. Convert 39.5 °C to Fahrenheit.

   (A) 103.1   (C) 103.3
   (B) 103.2   (D) 103.4

9. Convert 9:05 AM to military time.

   (A) 905   (C) 1905
   (B) 0905   (D) 2105

10. Convert 1829 to traditional time.

   (A) 8:29 AM   (C) 6:29 AM
   (B) 8:29 PM   (D) 6:29 PM

ANSWERS AND EXPLANATIONS

1. D

2. B

3. D

4. C

$$\frac{1{,}000\text{ mg}}{1\text{ g}} = \frac{x\text{ mg}}{0.75\text{ g}}$$

Cross multiply:

$$1{,}000 \times 0.75 = 1 \times x$$
$$750 = 1x$$
$$750 = x$$

Remember to label the answer correctly, in mg.

5. B

$$\frac{195\text{ lb}}{x\text{ kg}} = \frac{2.2\text{ lb}}{1\text{ kg}}$$

Cross multiply:

$$195 \times 1 = x \times 2.2$$
$$195 = 2.2x$$
$$88.63 = x$$

Label the answer with the correct units, kg.

6. D

$$\frac{30\text{ mL}}{1\text{ oz}} = \frac{x\text{ mL}}{4\text{ oz}}$$

Cross multiply:

$$30 \times 4 = 1 \times x$$
$$120 = 1x$$
$$120 = x$$

The answer is in mL.

7. C

$$(F - 32) \div 1.8 = \text{degrees Celsius}$$
$$(101.2 - 32) \div 1.8 = \text{degrees Celsius}$$
$$69.2 \div 1.8 = 38.4$$

8. A

$$(C \times 1.8) + 32 = \text{degrees Fahrenheit}$$
$$(39.5 \times 1.8) + 32 = 71.1$$
$$71.1 + 32 = 103.1$$

9. B

Delete the colon and the AM designation and add a zero (0) before the 9.

10. D

Subtract 1200 from 1829, leaving 629. Add the colon and the PM designation.

CHAPTER 8

Basic Problem Solving and Strategies for Dosage Calculation

The nurse can use several methods for calculating doses. Most nurses have a distinct preference regarding which method they use. Regardless of what method you feel most comfortable with, the end result, or answer, is the same from all three. The most common methods are the *ratio-proportion* and *formula* methods. Ratio-proportion was introduced in Chapter 5: Ratios and has been used up to this point in the text to solve for *x*. This chapter will introduce the formula method and help you to apply the ratio-proportion and formula methods to realistic clinical calculations.

A third method of calculating doses is called the *dimensional analysis* (DA) method. Dimensional analysis is a variation of the ratio-proportion method and is sometimes referred to as the *factor method*. This method will be introduced in this chapter as well. When you check your answers to the chapter quiz, you will note that all three methods can be used to solve each problem.

Medication orders are typically written in terms of quantity of medication to be administered, rather than number of tablets or specific volume (e.g., furosemide 40 mg po bid). Before calculating an appropriate dosage, the nurse must first be able to interpret the medication order. Once interpreted, the dosage is calculated using the strength (concentration) of the medication form available (e.g., furosemide 20 mg tablets). Medications are ordered this way so that the amount to be administered is always clear, regardless of what strength medication may be available in a given setting or at a particular time.

THE MEDICATION ORDER

Medications are ordered, or prescribed, by health care providers with prescriptive authority. Physicians, physicians' assistants, and nurse practitioners prescribe the majority of medications in the health care system, but other professionals such as dentists and chiropractors are authorized to prescribe certain medications as well.

A prescriber may order a medication by writing the order on paper, by giving it verbally to appropriate medical personnel, or by entering the medication order directly into the electronic health record. Written orders may be either given directly to a patient in the form of a prescription, scanned and sent to the pharmacy electronically, or faxed. Verbal orders may be given in person or over the telephone to an RN, pharmacist, or pharmacy technician.

Regardless of the method used to generate the order, the information required for a complete and concise medication is fairly consistent. All medication orders must contain the following:

- The patient's name, plus a second identifier such as date of birth or medical record number.
- Drug name. Generic names are always preferred, but trade (brand) names are acceptable.
- Dosage of medication to be given, preferably ordered in metric. Remember, medications written in grains (gr), minims (m), or drams (dr) *should always be clarified and reordered* in appropriate units.
- Route of the medication to be given. If no route is specified, contact the prescriber for clarification.
- Frequency or schedule of administration (e.g., daily, twice daily, at bedtime, every four hours, etc.).
- Indications, or special instructions related to the order. For example, PRN ("as needed") medications always require a reason (e.g., "as needed for pain" or "PRN sore throat").
- The date (including year) and time that the medication order was written or created.
- The prescriber's signature, either written or electronic.

> **Math Tip:** When in doubt, write it out! Avoid using abbreviations that could be confusing or ambiguous. It is much safer to write out the information than to use an abbreviation that could result in a medication error.

Each facility has an approved abbreviation list. Standard abbreviations are used to describe dosages, drug forms, routes, and times of administration.

The Joint Commission (TJC) requires that each facility develop an approved abbreviation list for staff and physicians to use. TJC has also developed a list of abbreviations that should not be used, as they have been known to result in medication errors.

If a medication order contains an abbreviation or other information that is unclear, always contact the prescriber for clarification before proceeding.

UNACCEPTABLE ABBREVIATIONS

In an effort to reduce errors in interpretation of medical abbreviations and symbols, in 2004 the Joint Commission began to require its member hospitals and outpatient centers to avoid the use of certain abbreviations that were previously acceptable. The following table lists terms that must be written out completely to prevent medical errors.

Abbreviation	Potential Problem	Preferred Term
U (for unit)	Mistaken as zero, 4, or cc.	Write "unit."
IU (for international unit)	Mistaken as IV (intravenous) or 10 (ten).	Write "international unit."
Q.D., QD, qd; Q.O.D., QOD, qod (Latin abbreviations for "once daily" and "every other day")	Mistaken for each other. The period after the Q can be mistaken for an I, and the O can be mistaken for I.	Write "daily" and "every other day."
Trailing zero (X.0 mg); lack of leading zero (.X mg)	Decimal point is missed.	Never write a zero by itself after a decimal point (X mg), and always use a zero before a decimal point (0.X mg).
MS	Can mean morphine sulfate or magnesium sulfate.	Write "morphine sulfate" or "magnesium sulfate."
MSO_4 $MgSO_4$	Confused for one another.	

The following abbreviations should also be avoided.

Abbreviation	Potential Problem	Preferred Term
µg (microgram)	Mistaken for mg (milligrams), resulting in one thousand–fold overdose	Write "mcg."
HS, hs (half-strength, or Latin abbreviation for "bedtime")	Mistaken for either "half-strength" or "hour of sleep (at bedtime)." q.H.S. mistaken for "every hour." All can result in a dosing error.	Write out "half-strength" or "at bedtime."
T.I.W., TIW, tiw (three times a week)	Mistaken for "three times a day" or "twice weekly," resulting in an overdose.	Write "3 times weekly" or "three times weekly."
SC, SQ, sub q (subcutaneous)	Mistaken as SL for sublingual or "5 every."	Write "Sub-Q," "subQ," or "subcutaneously."
D/C (discharge)	Interpreted as "Discontinue whatever medications follow" (typically discharge meds).	Write "discharge."
cc (cubic centimeter)	Mistaken for U (units) when poorly written.	Write "mL" for milliliters.
AS, AD, AU (Latin abbreviations for left, right, or both ears); OS, OD, OU (Latin abbreviations for left, right, or both eyes)	Mistaken for each other (e.g., AS for OS, AD for OD, AU for OU, etc.).	Write "left ear," "right ear," or "both ears"; "left eye," "right eye," or "both eyes."

For the complete list of "do not use" medical abbreviations, including any updates, see the Joint Commission's website: *www.jointcommission.org/topics/patient_safety.aspx.*

In addition, the Institute for Safe Medication Practices (ISMP) has published a list of dangerous abbreviations relating to medication use that it recommends avoiding. It is available on the ISMP website: *www.ismp.org.*

It is important for nurses to be familiar with their facility's policies and procedures regarding acceptable abbreviations.

INTERPRETING MEDICATION ORDERS

After a prescriber writes a medication order, that order must be interpreted before the proper medication form is chosen and the medication is administered. Consider the following order and its corresponding interpretation:

Furosemide 40 mg po bid

Drug name: *furosemide*

Dose: *40 mg*

Route: *oral (po)*

Frequency: *twice daily (bid)*

Practice 1

1. Interpret the following medication order:

   Amoxicillin suspension 250 mg po qid

   Drug name:

   Dose:

   Route:

   Frequency:

2. Interpret the following medication order:

   Lisinopril 10 mg po qhs

   Drug name:

   Dose:

   Route:

   Frequency:

3. Interpret the following medication order:

   Morphine sulfate 15 mg IM q 4 h prn pain

   Drug name:

   Dose:

   Route:

   Frequency:

   Indication:

UNDERSTANDING DRUG LABELS

The drug label contains information essential to administering an accurate dose of the medication. The drug label contains the following information:

- The drug name (generic and brand or trade name)

- The dosage strength, such as 125 mg/mL or 40 mg per tablet

- The route of administration, such as an oral liquid or a solution for injection

- Form of the drug, such as tablet, capsule, suppository, or ointment

- The total volume in the container for liquid medications or the number of tablets in the bottle

- Directions for mixing or reconstituting a medication

- Expiration date, manufacturer's name, National Drug Code (NDC) number, and precautions such as "protect from light"

In order to calculate accurately the amount of medication to be given, the nurse must know the dosage strength on hand.

For example, say the order is for "acetaminophen 650 mg po qid" and the drug label indicates that the bottle contains acetaminophen 325 mg tablets.

Obviously, the dose in the order and the dose available are not the same. This is when the ability to calculate a dose accurately is needed. It is simple for the nurse to look at the order and the drug label and know to administer two tablets for the patient to receive the correct dose. While this is a very basic calculation, many calculations are more complex.

> **Math Tip:** All three methods of calculating drug dosages require the nurse to know the same basic information. First, identify the drug dose ordered by the physician. Second, identify the dose available based on the drug label. Finally, identify the form and amount in which the drug comes (tablet, capsule, liquid).

USE OF RATIO-PROPORTION IN CALCULATING DOSES

Ratio-proportion is easy to use in dosage calculation. To set up the problem, first state the known ratio (325 mg : 1 tablet). This is the information that is available or is provided on the drug label. Then state the unknown ratio (650 mg : x tablets). Remember to label all terms of the ratios in the proportion, including x. Before solving the problem, estimate the answer.

For example, say the order is for "acetaminophen 650 mg po qid" and the drug label indicates that the bottle contains acetaminophen 325 mg tablets.

$$\underline{\text{Known} \qquad\qquad \text{Unknown or Desired}}$$
$$325 \text{ mg} : 1 \text{ tablet} \quad :: \quad 650 \text{ mg} : x \text{ tablets}$$

Simplify the problem by eliminating all the units, leaving only the numerals and the unknown, x.

$$325 : 1 :: 650 : x$$

Remember (from Chapter 5) that the double colon reads as "as" in the problem and functions as an equal sign. To solve for x, find the product of the extremes ($325 \times x = 325x$) and the product of the means ($1 \times 650 = 650$).

$325x = 650$ is the equation.

Divide both sides by the number in front of x, in this problem 325.

$$\frac{325x}{325} = \frac{650}{325}$$
$$x = 2$$

The nurse would administer two tablets for the correct dosage.

This problem can also be stated in a fraction format.

$$\underline{\text{Known} \qquad\qquad \text{Unknown or Desired}}$$
$$\frac{325 \text{ mg}}{1 \text{ tablet}} = \frac{600 \text{ mg}}{x \text{ tablets}}$$

To solve, cross multiply.

$$325 \times x = 1 \times 650$$
$$325x = 650$$

Divide both sides by the number in front of x, 325.

$$\frac{325x}{325} = \frac{650}{325}$$
$$x = 2$$

The nurse would administer two tablets for the correct dosage.

Two tablets is a logical dose. If the dosage were not logical—for example, if it indicated that the nurse should administer 20 tablets—that would suggest that the calculation was not correctly performed and should be set up and solved again. Remember to label the units of the answer, in this case "tablets."

> **Math Tip:** When using ratio-proportion in dosage calculation, state the units of measure in the same sequence. In this example, mg : tablet :: mg : tablet. Make sure that all terms are in the same units and system of measurement before setting up the problem. If they are not, you must complete that conversion before calculating the dose.

When solving a drug calculation problem, don't be confused by the name of the medication. The calculation itself is a mathematical equation and should be solved as such. If necessary, go back to Chapter 5 and review ratios before moving on in this chapter.

Practice 2

Solve the following problems using the ratio-proportion method. To make the problems easier for you, the drug names have been omitted.

1. The patient is to receive 15 mg of a drug. The tablets available are 10 mg tablets. How many tablets should be administered?

2. The patient is to receive 0.5 g of a drug. The drug is available in a 250 mg/5 mL solution. How much medication should be administered?

THE FORMULA METHOD

The formula method requires you to replace the terms in the formula with information from the problem. It can be used when calculating doses within the same units of measurement. If the dose desired and the dose available (on hand) are in different systems, they must be converted to the same units before solving the problem.

The formula is written as follows:

$$\frac{D}{H} \times Q = x$$

D stands for the *desired* dose, or the dose as ordered by the physician. It should include the weight, such as g, mg, etc.

H represents the dosage strength available, or the dose *on hand*. It should include the weight, such as g, mg, etc.

Q is the *quantity*, or the unit of measure, that contains the dose available or the number of capsules, milliliters, etc., that contains the available dosage.

> **Math Tip:** You may have learned a slightly different version of the formula. Some nurses use *V* for *vehicle*, rather than *Q*, when setting up the formula. The end result or answer is the same.

For example, say the order is for 40 mg of the drug. The label indicates that the drug is available in 10 mg/mL. How many mL of the medication should be administered?

Begin by inserting the numbers in the problem into the formula.

$$\frac{D \,(40\ \text{mg})}{H \,(10\ \text{mg})} \times Q\,(1\ \text{mL}) = x$$

Now that your problem is set up, eliminate the symbols from the formula (*D*, *H*, and *Q*) to leave only your unknown, *x*. Cancel out the units that appear in both the numerator and denominator, and solve the problem.

$$\frac{40 \times 1}{10} \ \text{ or } \ \frac{40}{10} \ \text{ or } \ 4\ \text{mL} = x$$

The nurse would administer 4 mL of the drug.

> **Math Tip:** Estimate a logical answer before solving the problem. Remember to label your answer correctly.

Practice 3

Solve the following problems using the formula method.

1. The order is for 75 mg of medication. The label indicates that each capsule contains 25 mg. How many capsules should be administered?

2. The order is for 1 g of medication. The label indicates that each tablet contains 1,000 mg. How many tablets should be administered?

3. The order is for 0.55 g of medication. The label indicates that each mL of the drug contains 250 mg. How many mL should be administered?

DIMENSIONAL ANALYSIS

Dimensional analysis is an easy, commonsense approach to dosage calculations that eliminates the need to remember a formula. Dimensional analysis is also known as *factor analysis* or *factor labeling*. While the term itself may be intimidating, many nurses find dimensional analysis to be the simplest manner of performing a dosage calculation. Solving a problem with dimensional analysis involves six steps:

1. Identify the *given* quantity in the problem.

2. Identify the *wanted* quantity or answer to the problem—this is the unknown or *x*.

3. Identify the *equivalents* involved in the problem.

4. *Set up* the problem, using equivalents as conversion factors.

5. *Cancel the units* that appear in both the numerator and the denominator to determine the unit of your unknown.

6. *Multiply* the numerators, *multiply* the denominators, and *divide* the product of the numerators by the product of the denominators to find the answer.

For example, suppose you want to convert 15 ounces into milliliters. Some problems contain all of the information that you need. Other problems will require an additional conversion factor. In this problem, you will need to use the common conversion factor of 1 ounce = 30 mL.

STEP 1: Identify the given quantity in the problem.

15 ounces

STEP 2: Identify the wanted quantity, or answer to the problem. At this time, it is unknown.

x mL

STEP 3: Identify the equivalents involved in the problem. In this case, there is one equivalent relationship.

1 ounce = 30 mL

STEP 4: Set up the problem using equivalents as conversion factors. Always start by setting up the given quantity over a denominator of 1. Then, make sure the units of measurement you want to cancel out appear in both the numerator and denominator.

$$\frac{15 \text{ oz}}{1} \times \frac{30 \text{ mL}}{1 \text{ oz}}$$

STEP 5: Cancel the units that appear in both the numerator and the denominator to determine the unit of your unknown, or x.

$$\frac{15}{1} \times \frac{30 \text{ mL}}{1}$$

Here, the unit of your unknown quantity is mL.

STEP 6: Multiply the numerators, multiply the denominators, and divide the product of the numerators by the product of the denominators to find the answer.

$15 \times 30 = 450$ (multiply the numerators)
$1 \times 1 = 1$ (multiply the denominators)
450 (divide the products)

There are 450 mL in 15 ounces.

Often the only equivalent relationship that you need is provided in the problem. However, when quantities are given in different units of measurement, you must convert one in order to perform your calculation accurately. To accomplish this, more equivalents can be added to the dimensional analysis equation.

For example, the order is for Kanamycin 1 g po. The label indicates that each capsule contains 500 mg of medication. How many capsules should be administered?

STEP 1: Identify the given quantity in the problem.

1 g

STEP 2: Identify the wanted quantity or answer to the problem. At this time, it is unknown.

x capsules

STEP 3: Identify the equivalents involved in the problem. One equivalent relationship is provided in the problem. Because the given quantity (1 g) and the dosage strength (500 mg) are in different units, you must also include the equivalent relationship between these units.

1 capsule = 500 mg
1,000 mg = 1 g

STEP 4: Set up the problem, using equivalents as conversion factors. Start by setting up the given quantity over a denominator of 1. Make sure the units you want to cancel out appear in both the numerator and denominator.

$$\frac{1 \text{ g}}{1} \times \frac{1,000 \text{ mg}}{1 \text{ g}} \times \frac{1 \text{ capsule}}{500 \text{ mg}}$$

STEP 5: Cancel the units that appear in both the numerator and the denominator to determine the unit of the unknown quantity.

$$\frac{1}{1} \times \frac{1,000}{1} \times \frac{1 \text{ capsule}}{500}$$

STEP 6: Multiply the numerators, multiply the denominators, and divide the product of the numerators by the product of the denominators to find the answer.

$$
\begin{array}{ll}
1 \times 1,000 \times 1 = 1,000 & \text{(multiply the numerators)} \\
1 \times 1 \times 500 = \overline{500} & \text{(multiply the denominators)} \\
\qquad\qquad\qquad 2 & \text{(divide the products)}
\end{array}
$$

You should administer two capsules.

Practice 4

Solve the following problems using dimensional analysis.

1. The order is for 50 mg of the drug. The label indicates that the drug is available in 20 mg/mL. How many mL of the drug should be administered?

2. The order is for 250 mg of the drug. The label indicates that the drug is available in 100 mg/mL. How many mL of the drug should be administered?

3. The order is for 0.75 g of the drug. The label indicates that the drug is available in 1,200 mg/120 mL. How many mL of the drug should be administered?

Most nurses find that they prefer one method over the others. Since all three methods can be used to calculate dosages accurately, which one to use is a matter of personal preference. Most nurses will continue to calculate dosages using the method they were taught when they were first introduced to dosage calculations. However, it is a good exercise to practice calculating dosages using the other two methods; you can deepen your understanding of the relationships of units of measurement and use one method to double-check another. You will build on the basic problem-solving skills you learned in this chapter and apply them to oral medications, parenteral medications, IV medications, and pediatric doses in Chapters 9–12.

ANSWERS AND EXPLANATIONS TO PRACTICE EXERCISES

Practice 1

1.

The name of the drug to be given is **amoxicillin suspension**.

The dose required is **250 mg**.

The desired route of administration is **oral** (po).

The frequency of administration is **four times daily** (qid).

2.

The name of the drug to be given is **lisinopril**.

The dose required is **10 mg**.

The desired route of administration is **oral**.

The frequency of administration is **nightly at bedtime** (qhs).

3.

The name of the drug to be given is **morphine sulfate**.

The dose required is **15 mg**.

The desired route of administration is **IM**.

The frequency of administration is **every four hours as needed for pain**.

Practice 2

1. 1.5 or $1\frac{1}{2}$ tablets

$$\frac{\text{Known}}{10\,\text{mg}:1\,\text{tablet}} \because \frac{\text{Unknown}}{15\,\text{mg}:x\,\text{tablets}}$$

Multiply the means and the extremes.

$$10x \because 15$$

Divide both sides of the proportion by the number in front of x, 10.

$$x = 1.5 \text{ or } 1\frac{1}{2} \text{ tablets.}$$

2. 10 mL

In this calculation, the unit of measurement in the order (0.5 g) and the unit of measurement on the label (250 mg/5 mL) are not the same.

Begin by converting 0.5 g to 500 mg. Then solve the problem.

$$\frac{\text{Known}}{250\,\text{mg}:5\,\text{mL}} \because \frac{\text{Unknown}}{500\,\text{mg}:x\,\text{mL}}$$

Multiply the means and the extremes.

$$250x \because 2{,}500$$

Divide both sides of the proportion by the number in front of x, 250.

$$x = 10 \text{ mL}$$

Practice 3

1. 3 capsules

Begin by inserting the numbers in the problem into the formula.

$$\frac{D\,(75\,\text{mg})}{H\,(25\,\text{mg})} \times Q\,(1\text{ capsule}) = x$$

Cancel out the units that appear in both the numerator and the denominator, and solve the problem.

$$\frac{75 \times 1}{25} \text{ or } \frac{75}{25} \text{ or 3 capsules} = x$$

2. 1 tablet

Begin by converting 1 g into 1,000 mg. Then insert the numbers in the problem into the formula.

$$\frac{D\,(1{,}000\,\text{mg})}{H\,(1{,}000\,\text{mg})} \times Q\,(1\text{ capsule}) = x$$

Cancel out the units that appear in both the numerator and the denominator, and solve the problem.

$$\frac{1{,}000 \times 1}{1{,}000} \text{ or } \frac{1{,}000}{1{,}000} \text{ or 1 tablet} = x$$

3. 2.2 mL

Begin converting 0.55 g into 550 mg. Then insert the numbers in the problem into the formula.

$$\frac{D\ (550\ mg)}{H\ (250\ mg)} \times Q\ (1\ mL) = x$$

Cancel out the units that appear in both the numerator and the denominator, and solve the problem.

$$\frac{550 \times 1}{250} \text{ or } \frac{550}{250} \text{ or } 2.2\ mL = x$$

Practice 4

1. 2.5 mL

STEP 1: Identify the given quantity in the problem.

50 mg

STEP 2: Identify the wanted quantity or answer to the problem—at this time, it is unknown.

x mL

STEP 3: Identify the equivalents involved in the problem. Since the given quantity and the dosage strength are in the same units, the only equivalent that you need is the one provided in the problem.

20 mg = 1 mL

STEP 4: Set up the problem using equivalents as conversion factors. Start by setting up the given quantity over a denominator of 1. Make sure the units you want to cancel out appear in both the numerator and denominator.

$$\frac{50\ mg}{1} \times \frac{1\ mL}{20\ mg}$$

STEP 5: Cancel the units that appear in both the numerator and the denominator to determine the unit of your unknown quantity.

$$\frac{50}{1} \times \frac{1\ mL}{20}$$

STEP 6: Multiply the numerators, multiply the denominators, and divide the product of the numerators by the product of the denominators to find the answer.

$$\begin{array}{ll} 50 \times 1 = \underline{50} & \text{(multiply the numerators)} \\ 1 \times 20 = \overline{20} & \text{(multiply the denominators)} \\ \quad\quad\ 2.5 & \text{(divide the products)} \end{array}$$

2. 2.5 mL

STEP 1: Identify the given quantity in the problem.

250 mg

STEP 2: Identify the wanted quantity, or answer to the problem. At this time, it is unknown.

x mL

STEP 3: Identify the equivalents involved in the problem. Since the given quantity and the dosage strength are in the same units, the only equivalent that you need is provided in the problem.

100 mg = 1 mL

STEP 4: Set up the problem, using equivalents as conversion factors. Start by setting up the given quantity over a denominator of 1. Make sure the units you want to cancel out appear in both the numerator and denominator.

$$\frac{250\ mg}{1} \times \frac{1\ mL}{100\ mg}$$

STEP 5: Cancel the units that appear in both the numerator and the denominator to determine the unit of x.

$$\frac{250}{1} \times \frac{1\ mL}{100}$$

STEP 6: Multiply the numerators, multiply the denominators, and divide the product of the numerators by the product of the denominators to find the answer.

$$\begin{array}{ll} 250 \times 1 = \underline{250} & \text{(multiply the numerators)} \\ 1 \times 100 = \overline{100} & \text{(multiply the denominators)} \\ \quad\quad\quad\ 2.5 & \text{(divide the products)} \end{array}$$

3. 75 mL

STEP 1: Identify the given quantity in the problem.

0.75 g

STEP 2: Identify the wanted quantity, or answer to the problem. At this time, it is unknown.

x mL

STEP 3: Identify the equivalents involved in the problem. One equivalent relationship is provided. Since the given quantity (0.75 g) and the dosage strength (1,200 mg) are in different units, you must also include the equivalent relationship between these units.

1,200 mg = 120 mL

1 g = 1,000 mg

STEP 4: Set up the problem using equivalents as conversion factors. Start by setting up the given quantity over a denominator of 1. Make sure the units you want to cancel out appear in both the numerator and denominator.

$$\frac{0.75 \text{ g}}{1} \times \frac{1,000 \text{ mg}}{1 \text{ g}} \times \frac{120 \text{ mL}}{1,200 \text{ mg}}$$

STEP 5: Cancel the units that appear in both the numerator and the denominator to determine the unit of the unknown quantity.

$$\frac{0.75}{1} \times \frac{1,000}{1} \times \frac{120 \text{ mL}}{1,200}$$

STEP 6: Multiply the numerators, multiply the denominators, and divide the product of the numerators by the product of the denominators to find the answer.

$$
\begin{array}{ll}
0.75 \times 1,000 \times 120 = \underline{90,000} & \text{(multiply the numerators)} \\
1 \times 1 \times 1,200 = 1,200 & \text{(multiply the denominators)} \\
75 & \text{(divide the products)}
\end{array}
$$

CHAPTER QUIZ

Solve each of the problems using the method you prefer. All three methods are included in the chapter quiz answers and explanations.

1. The order is for Furosemide 80 mg. The drug available is Furosemide 40 mg/5 mL solution. How much should be administered?

   (A) 0.5 mL   (C) 5 mL

   (B) 1.5 mL   (D) 10 mL

2. The order is for Meperedine 35 mg. The drug available is Meperedine 100 mg/1 mL solution. How much should be administered?

   (A) 0.35 mL   (C) 35 mL

   (B) 3.5 mL   (D) 350 mL

3. The order is for Aspirin 325 mg. The drug available is Aspirin 81 mg/tablet. How much should be administered?

   (A) 2 tablets   (C) 4 tablets

   (B) 3 tablets   (D) 5 tablets

4. The order is for KCL 20 mEq. The drug available is KCL 60 mEq/15 mL solution. How much should be administered?

    (A) 3 mL   (C) 10 mL

    (B) 5 mL   (D) 30 mL

5. The order is for Amoxicillin 300 mg. The drug available is Amoxicillin 250 mg/5 mL suspension. How much should be administered?

    (A) 2 mL   (C) 6 mL

    (B) 4 mL   (D) 8 mL

6. The order is for Penicillin 250,000 units. The drug available is Penicillin 1,000,000 units/5 mL solution. How much should be administered?

    (A) 1.25 mL   (C) 4.85 mL

    (B) 3.75 mL   (D) 6.25 mL

7. The order is for Dexamethasone 0.75 mg. The drug available is Dexamethasone 0.25 mg/tablet. How much should be administered?

   (A) 0.3 tablets (C) 2 tablets

   (B) 1.5 tablets (D) 3 tablets

8. The order is for Cimetidine 0.4 g. The drug available is Cimetidine 400 mg/tablet. How much should be administered?

   (A) 0.4 tablets (C) 4 tablets

   (B) 1 tablet (D) 10 tablets

9. The order is for Digoxin 0.5 mg. The drug available is Digoxin 0.125 mg/tablet. How much should be administered?

   (A) 2 tablets   (C) 4 tablets
   (B) 3 tablets   (D) 5 tablets

10. The order is for Atropine sulfate 0.6 mg. The drug available is Atropine sulfate 0.4 mg/mL solution. How much should be administered?

    (A) 1.5 mL   (C) 2.5 mL
    (B) 2 mL   (D) 3 mL

ANSWERS AND EXPLANATIONS

The answers and explanations for this chapter quiz show all three methods to solve the problems.

1. D

Ratio-proportion method

40 mg : 5 mL :: 80 mg : x mL

Multiply the means and the extremes:
40x = 400 is the equation.

Divide both sides by the number in front of x,
40: x = 10.

Formula method

$$\frac{D\,(80\text{ mg})}{H\,(40\text{ mg})} \times Q\,(5\text{ mL}) = x$$

$$\frac{80 \times 5}{40} \text{ or } \frac{400}{40} \text{ or } 10\text{ mL} = x$$

$$x = 10$$

Dimensional analysis

Identify the given quantity (80 mg), the wanted quantity (x mL), and the equivalents involved (40 mg = 5 mL). Set up the problem, starting with the given quantity over a denominator of 1.

$$\frac{80\text{ mg}}{1} \times \frac{5\text{ mL}}{40\text{ mg}}$$

$$\frac{80}{1} \times \frac{5\text{ mL}}{40}$$

80 × 5 = 400 (multiply the numerators)
1 × 40 = 40 (multiply the denominators)
10 (divide the products)

Administer 10 mL.

2. A

Ratio-proportion method

100 mg : 1 mL :: 35 mg : x mL

Multiply the means and the extremes:
100x = 35 is the equation.

Divide both sides by the number in front of x,
100: x = 0.35.

Formula method

$$\frac{D\,(35\text{ mg})}{H\,(100\text{ mg})} \times Q\,(1\text{ mL}) = x$$

$$\frac{35 \times 1}{100} \text{ or } \frac{35}{100} \text{ or } 0.35\text{ mL} = x$$

Dimensional analysis

Identify the given quantity (35 mg), the wanted quantity (x mL), and the equivalents involved (100 mg = 1 mL).

$$\frac{35\text{ mg}}{1} \times \frac{1\text{ mL}}{100\text{ mg}}$$

$$\frac{35}{1} \times \frac{1\text{ mL}}{100}$$

35 × 1 = 35 (multiply the numerators)
1 × 100 = 100 (multiply the denominators)
0.35 (divide the products)

Administer 0.35 mL.

3. C

Ratio-proportion method

81 mg : 1 tablet :: 325 mg : x tablets

Multiply the means and the extremes:
81x = 325 is the equation.

Divide both sides by the number in front of x,
81: x = 4.01

Formula method

$$\frac{D\,(325\text{ mg})}{H\,(81\text{ mg})} \times Q\,(1\text{ tablet}) = x$$

$$\frac{325 \times 1}{81} \text{ or } \frac{325}{81} \text{ or } 4.01\text{ tablets} = x$$

Dimensional analysis

Identify the given quantity (325 mg), the wanted quantity (x tablets), and the equivalents involved (81 mg = 1 tablet).

$$\frac{325\text{ mg}}{1} \times \frac{1\text{ tablet}}{81\text{ mg}}$$

$$\frac{325}{1} \times \frac{1\text{ tablet}}{81}$$

325 × 1 = 325 (multiply the numerators)
1 × 81 = 81 (multiply the denominators)
4.01 (divide the products)

Administer 4 tablets.

4. B

Ratio-proportion method

60 mEq : 15 mL :: 20 mEq : x mL

Multiply the means and the extremes: $60x = 300$ is the equation.

Divide both sides by the number in front of x, 60: $x = 5$.

Formula method

$$\frac{D\,(20\ \text{mEq})}{H\,(60\ \text{mEq})} \times Q\,(15\ \text{mL}) = x$$

$$\frac{20 \times 15}{60} \quad \text{or} \quad \frac{300}{60} \quad \text{or } 5\ \text{mL} = x$$

Dimensional analysis

Identify the given quantity (20 mEq), the wanted quantity (x mL), and the equivalents involved (60 mEq = 15 mL).

$$\frac{20\ \text{mEq}}{1} \times \frac{15\ \text{mL}}{60\ \text{mEq}}$$

$$\frac{20}{1} \times \frac{15\ \text{mL}}{60}$$

$20 \times 15 = \underline{300}$ (multiply the numerators)
$1 \times 60 = 60$ (multiply the denominators)
5 (divide the products)

Administer 5 mL.

5. C

Ratio-proportion method

250 mg : 5 mL :: 300 mg : x mL

Multiply the means and the extremes: $250x = 1,500$ is the equation.

Divide both sides by the number in front of x, 250: $x = 6$.

Formula method

$$\frac{D\,(300\ \text{mg})}{H\,(250\ \text{mg})} \times Q\,(5\ \text{mL}) = x$$

$$\frac{300 \times 5}{250} \quad \text{or} \quad \frac{1,500}{250} \quad \text{or } 6\ \text{mL} = x$$

Dimensional analysis

Identify the given quantity (300 mg), the wanted quantity (x mL), and the equivalents involved (250 mg = 5 mL).

$$\frac{300\ \text{mg}}{1} \times \frac{5\ \text{mL}}{250\ \text{mg}}$$

$$\frac{300}{1} \times \frac{5\ \text{mL}}{250}$$

$300 \times 5 = \underline{1,500}$ (multiply the numerators)
$1 \times 250 = 250$ (multiply the denominators)
6 (divide the products)

Administer 6 mL.

6. A

Ratio-proportion method

1,000,000 units : 5 mL :: 250,000 units : x mL

Multiply the means and the extremes: $1,000,000x = 1,250,000$ is the equation.

Divide both sides by the number in front of x, 1,000,000: $x = 1.25$.

Formula method

$$\frac{D\,(250,000\ \text{units})}{H\,(1,000,000\ \text{units})} \times Q\,(5\ \text{mL}) = x$$

$$\frac{250,000 \times 5}{1,000,000} \quad \text{or} \quad \frac{1,250,000}{1,000,000} \quad \text{or } 1.25\ \text{mL} = x$$

Dimensional analysis

Identify the given quantity (250,000 units), the wanted quantity (x mL), and the equivalents involved (1,000,000 units = 5 mL).

$$\frac{250,000\ \text{units}}{1} \times \frac{5\ \text{mL}}{1,000,000\ \text{units}}$$

$$\frac{250,000}{1} \times \frac{5\ \text{mL}}{1,000,000}$$

$250,000 \times 5 = \underline{1,250,000}$ (multiply the numerators)
$1 \times 1,000,000 = \overline{1,000,000}$ (multiply the denominators)
1.25 (divide the products)

Administer 1.25 mL.

7. D

Ratio-proportion method

0.25 mg : 1 tablet :: 0.75 mg : x tablets

Multiply the means and the extremes: $0.25x = 0.75$ is the equation.

Divide both sides by the number in front of x, $0.25 : x = 3$.

Formula method

$$\frac{D\,(0.75\text{ mg})}{H\,(0.25\text{ mg})} \times Q\,(1\text{ tablet}) = x$$

$$\frac{0.75 \times 1}{0.25} \quad \text{or} \quad \frac{0.75}{0.25} \quad \text{or 3 tablets} = x$$

Dimensional analysis

Identify the given quantity (0.75 mg), the wanted quantity (x tablets), and the equivalents involved (0.25 mg = 1 tablet).

$$\frac{0.75\text{ mg}}{1} \times \frac{1\text{ tablet}}{0.25\text{ mg}}$$

$$\frac{0.75}{1} \times \frac{1\text{ tablet}}{0.25}$$

0.75 × 1 = 0.75 (multiply the numerators)
1 × 0.25 = 2.50 (multiply the denominators)
          3   (divide the products)

Administer 3 tablets.

8. B

Ratio-proportion method

Since the known and the unknown are in different units of measurement, convert 0.4 g into 400 mg before continuing to solve the problem.

400 mg : 1 tablet :: 400 mg : x tablets

Multiply the means and the extremes: $400x = 400$ is the equation.

Divide both sides by the number in front of x, $400 : x = 1$.

Once the conversion is completed, it should not be necessary to continue with the calculation, as the correct answer is obvious.

Formula method

Since the dose desired (D) and the dosage strength on hand (H) are in different units of measurement, convert 0.4 g into 400 mg before continuing to solve the problem.

$$\frac{D\,(400\text{ mg})}{H\,(400\text{ mg})} \times Q\,(1\text{ tablet}) = x$$

$$\frac{400 \times 1}{400} \quad \text{or} \quad \frac{400}{400} \quad \text{or 1 tablet} = x$$

Dimensional analysis

Identify the given quantity (0.4 g), the wanted quantity (x tablets), and the equivalents involved (400 mg = 1 tablet, and 1,000 mg = 1 g).

$$\frac{0.4\text{ g}}{1} \times \frac{1{,}000\text{ mg}}{1\text{ g}} \times \frac{1\text{ tablet}}{0.4\text{ mg}}$$

$$\frac{0.4}{1} \times \frac{1{,}000}{1} \times \frac{1\text{ tablet}}{0.4}$$

0.4 × 1,000 × 1 = 0.4 (multiply the numerators)
  1 × 1 × 0.4 = 0.4 (multiply the denominators)
              1   (divide the products)

Administer 1 tablet.

9. C

Ratio-proportion method

0.125 mg : 1 tablet :: 0.5 mg : x tablets

Multiply the means and the extremes:
$0.125x = 0.5$ is the equation.

Divide both sides by the number in front of x,
$0.125 : x = 4$.

Formula method

$$\frac{D\ (0.5\ \text{mg})}{H\ (0.125\ \text{mg})} \times Q\ (1\ \text{tablet}) = x$$

$$\frac{0.5 \times 1}{0.125} \quad \text{or} \quad \frac{0.5}{0.125} \quad \text{or 4 tablets} = x$$

Dimensional analysis

Identify the given quantity (0.5 mg),
the wanted quantity (x tablets), and the
equivalents involved (0.125 mg = 1 tablet).

$$\frac{0.5\ \text{mg}}{1} \times \frac{1\ \text{tablet}}{0.125\ \text{mg}}$$

$$\frac{0.5}{1} \times \frac{1\ \text{tablet}}{0.125}$$

$0.5 \times 1 = \underline{0.5}$ (multiply the numerators)
$1 \times 0.125 = \overline{0.125}$ (multiply the denominators)
            4 (divide the products)

Administer 4 tablets.

10. A

Ratio-proportion method

0.4 mg : 1 mL :: 0.6 mg : x mL

Multiply the means and the extremes:
$0.4x = 0.6$ is the equation.

Divide both sides by the number in front of x,
$0.4 : x = 1.5$.

Formula method

$$\frac{D\ (0.6\ \text{mg})}{H\ (0.4\ \text{mg})} \times Q\ (1\ \text{mL}) = x$$

$$\frac{0.6 \times 1}{0.4} \quad \text{or} \quad \frac{0.6}{0.4} \quad \text{or 1.5 mL} = x$$

Dimensional analysis

Identify the given quantity (0.6 mg), the
wanted quantity (x mL), and the equivalents
involved (0.4 mg = 1 mL).

$$\frac{0.6\ \text{mg}}{1} \times \frac{1\ \text{mL}}{0.4\ \text{mg}}$$

$$\frac{0.6}{1} \times \frac{1\ \text{mL}}{0.4}$$

$0.6 \times 1 = \underline{0.6}$ (multiply the numerators)
$1 \times 0.4 = \overline{0.4}$ (multiply the denominators)
        1.5 (divide the products)

Administer 1.5 mL.

CHAPTER 9

Oral Medications

Oral administration of medications is generally the easiest, most cost-effective, and most commonly used route of administration. The oral route of administration is referred to as PO or p.o., which is Latin for *per os*, meaning through the mouth.

Oral medications are available as tablets, capsules, caplets, liquids, and powders. While there are many advantages to oral administration, there are disadvantages as well. Some drugs, such as insulin, are inactivated by stomach acid and cannot be given orally. Gastric mucosa can be irritated by medications, resulting in nausea, vomiting, and ulceration. Some drugs are affected by certain foods and drinks, inhibiting the absorption rate or causing adverse side effects.

It is important to pay close attention to the medication label regarding any warnings or information pertaining to the route of administration. For example, a liquid medication may contain a warning indicating that it is for topical use only. Saturated solution of potassium iodide (SSKI) must be diluted in a glass of liquid, such as juice, prior to administration.

This chapter will describe the different forms of oral medications and cover the correct way to calculate their dosage.

DRUG FORMS

Before a drug receives final approval from the Food and Drug Administration (FDA), the drug company must indicate in what form or forms it will be manufactured. Some drugs are manufactured in several forms. For example, oral acetaminophen is available as a tablet, capsule, caplet, and liquid.

Capsule

Capsules come in a variety of shapes and sizes and are available in two varieties. The first type of capsule is a rigid gelatin shell manufactured in two pieces that fit together. It contains the drug in a powdered, granular, or pellet form. Many oral antibiotics are manufactured in this manner. Some rigid gelatin capsules can be opened and the powdered medication mixed with a soft food for patients who have difficulty swallowing. Other capsules contain sustained-release medications and should be administered whole to achieve the desired effect. Many over-the-counter cold preparations should not be opened or altered in any way.

The second type is a softer gelatin shell containing medication in liquid form. Stool softeners and fat-soluble vitamins may be manufactured in a soft shell. Capsules are available in a variety of colors, shapes, sizes, and dosage strengths.

Capsules cannot be divided, so a dose must include only whole capsules. The abbreviation *cap* or *caps* may be used to indicate a capsule form of a medication.

Liquids

Many medications are available in a liquid form. Liquid medications contain a specific amount, or weight, of medication in a given volume of liquid. This information is contained on the label. Some liquid medications come in several dosage strengths, so it is important to pay close attention to the label information when calculating a liquid dose.

Solutions contain a drug dissolved in a water base. Solutions do not need to be mixed, as the water-to-drug concentration is the same throughout the solution.

Syrups, such as over-the-counter cough preparations, are thick solutions containing medication, water, sugar, and flavoring.

Elixirs are thinner than syrups and contain alcohol, water, sugar, and flavoring in addition to the medication.

Suspensions, such as antacids, contain fine, undissolved particles of drug suspended in a water base. With prolonged standing, the particles gradually settle to the bottom and must be shaken to redistribute the medication prior to administration.

Artificial flavors such as grape, cherry, or bubblegum can be added to oral medications to make them more palatable. Liquids allow for a variety of doses and may be measured using droppers, syringes, medicine cups, or hollow-handled spoons.

Tablets

Tablets contain dried, powdered active drugs along with inert binders and fillers that allow them to be molded into various shapes and sizes. Tablets come in a range of varying doses, which should always be expressed in metric (grams, milligrams, or micrograms). Some tablets are scored to allow them to be broken into equal halves, thirds, or quarters. To ensure accurate dosing, tablets that are not scored should never be broken, and scored tablets should only be cut or broken along their score lines.

An enteric-coated tablet is covered with a special coating that is resistant to stomach acid to prevent stomach irritation. Instead, it dissolves in the alkaline environment of the small intestine. Enteric-coated tablets are not scored and should not be crushed or altered, as crushing destroys the protective coating and can result in stomach irritation or improper absorption.

Sustained-release (SR), extended-release (ER), or long-acting (LA) tablets are designed to provide a continuous release of the drug over a prolonged period of time. These tablets should never be crushed or chewed, which would cause them to be absorbed much more quickly than intended. Occasionally these tablets may be scored, so that they may be split. If a sustained-release, extended-release, or long-acting tablet is not scored, it is especially important that it never be cut or split.

Caplets are coated tablets that are manufactured in the shape of capsules. Some caplets can be crushed. However, others may contain sustained-release medications.

Some tablets, such as effervescent tablets for cold symptoms, are designed to be dissolved in water before being taken orally. Lozenges are round, flat tablets formed from a hardened sugar base that are designed to dissolve slowly in the mouth to release the drug. A troche is another type of tablet with a sugar base that releases medication as it dissolves in the mouth.

The abbreviation *tab* or *tabs* may be used to indicate a tablet form of a medication.

Powders

A powder is a finely ground form of an active drug. Powdered drugs (such as bulk laxatives) may be added to water immediately before administering. Some oral antibiotics are packaged as a powder that must be reconstituted with a specific amount of diluent prior to administration. Information regarding appropriate liquids to use as a diluent is included on the drug label.

CALCULATING DOSES OF TABLETS AND CAPSULES

The ratio-proportion, formula, or dimensional analysis method may be used to calculate doses of tablets and capsules. Regardless of which method you prefer, make sure to double-check your calculations before administering the medication. Doses should be logical. If a calculation requires the nurse to give more than four tablets or capsules, the calculation may have been performed incorrectly, or a stronger strength of the medication may be desirable. Likewise, a calculation that would require you to give one half of a capsule or less than a full nonscored tablet would not be logical.

For example, the order is for Ibuprofen 800 mg. The label indicates that each tablet contains 200 mg of medication.

$$800 \text{ mg} : x \text{ tablets} :: 200 \text{ mg} : 1 \text{ tablet}$$
$$(\text{extremes}) \; 800 :: 200x \; (\text{means})$$
$$4 = x$$

Using ratio-proportion to solve this problem, the correct dose of this medication would be four tablets. Since ibuprofen is available in 200 mg, 400 mg, 600 mg, and 800 mg tablets, the patient may prefer to take one 800 mg tablet rather than four 200 mg tablets.

Even though the dose is equivalent, other factors may have to be considered. For example, 800 mg tablets are available only by prescription, while 200 mg tablets are available over-the-counter. This could affect the cost of the medication and be a consideration. Also, the 800 mg tablet of this particular medication is much larger than the 200 mg tablet and may be more difficult to swallow for some patients.

Typically with prescription medications, the physician will order the dose that requires the patient to take the smallest number of tablets. There has been a recent trend toward ordering scored tablets at a higher dose and instructing the patient to break the tablet in half as a cost-saving method. However, this method would not commonly be used in an institutional setting, as most facilities would not have the ability to store the remaining half-tablet for future use.

> **Math Tip:** Remember that correctly performing the math component of a dosage calculation does not mean that the nurse should proceed with giving the medication. Doses that exceed four tablets or capsules, are extremely large, or require a nonscored tablet to be altered should be clarified before proceeding.

Practice 1

Solve the following problems using the ratio-proportion method.

1. Order: Ciprofloxacin hydrochloride 500 mg PO BID
   Available: Ciprofloxacin hydrochloride 250 mg tablets
   How many tablets should be administered?

2. Order: Phenytoin 15 mg PO BID
   Available: Phenytoin 30 mg capsules
   How many capsules should be administered?

3. Order: Diltiazem CD 180 mg PO daily
   Available: Diltiazem SR 60 mg capsules
   How many capsules should be administered?

4. Order: Doxycycline 1,000 mg PO BID
   Available: Doxycycline 100 mg tablets
   How many tablets should be administered?

CALCULATING LIQUID MEDICATIONS

The ratio-proportion, formula, or dimensional analysis method may be used to calculate doses of liquid medications. Using a liquid form of a medication may be beneficial for pediatric patients; patients who have difficulty swallowing solid medications; or patients who receive their medications through a nasogastric, gastrostomy, or jejunostomy tube. Another benefit of using a liquid medication is that it allows for more options for dosing the drug. For example, amoxicillin is available in 250 mg and 500 mg capsules as well as 200 mg, 250 mg, 400 mg, and 500 mg tablets. Amoxicillin oral suspension is available in 125 mg/5 mL, 200 mg/5 mL, 250 mg/5 mL, and 400 mg/5 mL strengths. If the physician wants a pediatric patient to receive "Amoxicillin 300 mg PO every 8 hours," it would be impossible to administer that dose using capsules or tablets; however, it could be administered using the liquid suspension.

Example:

Order: Amoxicillin 300 mg PO every 8 hours

Available: Amoxicillin oral suspension 200 mg/5 mL

Using the formula method introduced in Chapter 8 ($\frac{D}{H} \times Q = x$), it is easy to calculate the correct dosage.

> **Math Tip:** Remember that when using the formula method, D stands for desired dose, H represents the dose available or on hand, and Q is the quantity or unit of measure that contains the dose available.

$$\frac{D\,(300\text{ mg})}{H\,(200\text{ mg})} \times Q\,(5\text{ mL}) = x$$

$$\frac{300 \times 5}{200} \text{ or } \frac{1,500}{200} \text{ or } 7.5\text{ mL} = x$$

The nurse would administer 7.5 mL of the amoxicillin suspension.

Practice 2

Solve the following problems using the formula method.

1. Order: KCL elixir 25 mEq PO BID
   Available: KCL elixir 30 mEq/15 mL
   How much should be administered?

2. Order: Chlorpheniramine Maleate syrup 1.5 mg PO BID
   Available: Chlorpheniramine Maleate syrup 1 mg/8 mL
   How much should be administered?

3. Order: Cefaclor oral suspension 250 mg PO TID
   Available: Cefaclor oral suspension 375 mg/5 mL
   How much should be administered?

4. Order: Nystatin oral suspension 125,000 units swish and swallow TID
   Available: Nystatin oral suspension 100,000 units/mL
   How much should be administered?

SPECIAL CONSIDERATIONS

Some medications are available in only one strength and do not require a dosage calculation. For example, milk of magnesia is ordered by volume rather than strength. A typical order for this medication would be "MOM 30 mL at bedtime." Another type of medication that does not require calculating a dosage would be a multivitamin, which is usually ordered as "Multivitamin tablet 1 PO daily."

In addition, the dosing information contained on many over-the-counter (OTC) medications, such as cough suppressants or expectorants, indicates that a specific volume of the medication be taken. Even though the label lists the strength of the medication, the instructions are printed in a manner that makes it easier for the patient to understand how much to take. For example, the normal adult dose of guaifenesin syrup printed on the label is "10 mL every four hours as needed." Another example of a medication that is ordered by volume is the bulk-forming laxative psyllium. A common order would be "Psyllium 1 tablespoon in 8 ounces of liquid PO BID."

USING DIMENSIONAL ANALYSIS TO CALCULATE ORAL MEDICATIONS

The dimensional analysis method can be used to calculate the correct dosage of oral tablets, capsules, or liquid medications. The method you choose to perform dosage calculations is a matter of personal preference. As you learned in Chapter 8, the correct answer can be obtained by any of the three methods as long as the problem is solved correctly.

Example:

> Order: Ampicillin oral suspension 0.3 g PO every 6 hours
> Available: Ampicillin oral suspension 100 mg/5 mL

STEP 1: Identify the given quantity in the problem.

> 0.3 g

STEP 2: Identify the wanted quantity or answer to the problem. At this time it is unknown.

> *x* mL

STEP 3: Identify the equivalents involved in the problem. One equivalent relationship is provided. Since the given quantity (0.3 g) and the dosage strength (100 mg) are in different units of measurement, you must also include the equivalent relationship between these units.

> 100 mg = 5 mL
> 1,000 mg = 1 g

STEP 4: Set up the problem using equivalents as conversion factors. Always start by setting up the given quantity over a denominator of 1. Make sure the units you want to cancel out appear in both the numerator and denominator.

$$\frac{0.3\text{ g}}{1} \times \frac{1{,}000\text{ g}}{1\text{ g}} \times \frac{5\text{ mL}}{100\text{ mg}}$$

STEP 5: Cancel the units that appear in both the numerator and the denominator to determine the unit of your answer.

$$\frac{0.3}{1} \times \frac{1{,}000}{1} \times \frac{5\text{ mL}}{100}$$

STEP 6: Multiply the numerators, multiply the denominators, and divide the product of the numerators by the product of the denominators to find the answer.

$$0.3 \times 1{,}000 \times 5 = \underline{1{,}500} \quad \text{(multiply the numerators)}$$
$$1 \times 1 \times 1\,00 = \;\;100 \quad \text{(multiply the denominators)}$$
$$\qquad\qquad\quad 15 \quad \text{(divide the products)}$$

Administer 15 mL of ampicillin oral suspension.

Practice 3

Solve the following problems using the dimensional analysis method.

1. Order: Sulfisoxazole 250 mg PO QID
    Available: Sulfisoxazole 0.5 g tablets
    How many tablets should be administered?

2. Order: Ibuprofen oral suspension 0.3 g PO every 6 hours prn pain
    Available: Ibuprofen oral suspension 100 mg/5 mL
    How much should be administered?

KAPLAN) NURSING

ANSWERS AND EXPLANATIONS TO PRACTICE EXERCISES

Practice 1

1. 2 tablets

500 mg : x tablets :: 250 mg :: 1 tablet
(extremes) 500 :: 250x (means)
2 = x

2. $\frac{1}{2}$ or 0.5

After completing this calculation, you can see that the nurse must administer 0.5 or $\frac{1}{2}$ capsule. Since a capsule cannot be broken in half, the appropriate action would be for the nurse to contact the physician regarding the order.

15 mg : x capsules :: 30 mg : 1 capsule
(extremes) 15 :: 30x (means)
0.5 = x

3. 0 capsules

Diltiazem CD is ordered, and Diltiazem SR is available and cannot be used. The nurse should contact the physician regarding the order.

4. 10 tablets

The answer is 10 tablets according to the calculation. However, 1,000 mg of this drug far exceeds the recommended dosage, and the order should be clarified with the physician before proceeding.

1,000 mg : x tablets :: 100 mg : 1 tablet
(extremes) 1,000 :: 100x (means)
10 = x

Practice 2

1. 12.5 mL

$$\frac{D\,(25\ \text{mEq})}{H\,(30\ \text{mEq})} \times Q\,(15\ \text{mL}) = x$$

$$\frac{25 \times 15}{30} \ \text{or} \ \frac{375}{30} \ \text{or } 12.5\ \text{mL} = x$$

2. 12 mL

$$\frac{D\,(1.5\ \text{mg})}{H\,(1\ \text{mg})} \times Q\,(8\ \text{mL}) = x$$

$$\frac{1.5 \times 8}{1} \ \text{or} \ \frac{12}{1} \ \text{or } 12\ \text{mL} = x$$

3. 3.3 mL

$$\frac{D\,(250\ \text{mg})}{H\,(375\ \text{mg})} \times Q\,(5\ \text{mL}) = x$$

$$\frac{250 \times 5}{375} \ \text{or} \ \frac{1,250}{375} \ \text{or } 3.3\ \text{mL} = x$$

4. 1.25 mL

$$\frac{D\,(125,000\ \text{units})}{H\,(100,000\ \text{units})} \times Q\,(1\ \text{mL}) = x$$

$$\frac{125,000 \times 1}{100,000} \ \text{or} \ \frac{125,000}{100,000} \ \text{or } 1.25\ \text{mL} = x$$

Practice 3

1. 0.5 or $\frac{1}{2}$ tablet (if the tablet is scored)

STEP 1: Identify the given quantity in the problem.

250 mg

STEP 2: Identify the wanted quantity, or answer to the problem. At this time it is unknown.

x tablets

STEP 3: Identify the equivalents involved in the problem. One equivalent relationship is provided. Since the given quantity (0.5 g) and the dosage strength (250 mg) are in different units, you must also include the equivalent relationship between these units.

0.5 g = 1 tablet
1,000 mg = 1 g

STEP 4: Set up the problem using equivalents as conversion factors. Start by setting up the given quantity over a denominator of 1. Make sure the units you want to cancel out appear in both the numerator and denominator.

$$\frac{250 \text{ mg}}{1} \times \frac{1 \text{ g}}{1,000 \text{ mg}} \times \frac{1 \text{ tablet}}{0.5 \text{ mg}}$$

STEP 5: Cancel the units that appear in both the numerator and the denominator to determine the unit of your unknown quantity.

$$\frac{250}{1} \times \frac{1}{1,000} \times \frac{1 \text{ tablet}}{0.5}$$

STEP 6: Multiply the numerators, multiply the denominators, and divide the product of the numerators by the product of the denominators to find the answer.

$250 \times 1 \times 1 = \underline{250}$ (multiply the numerators)
$1 \times 1,000 \times 0.5 = \overline{500}$ (multiply the denominators)
0.5 (divide the products)

Administer 0.5 or $\frac{1}{2}$ tablet (if the tablet is scored).

2. 15 mL

STEP 1: Identify the given quantity in the problem.

0.3 g

STEP 2: Identify the wanted quantity or answer to the problem. At this time, it is unknown.

x mL

STEP 3: Identify the equivalents involved in the problem. One equivalent relationship is provided. Since the given quantity (0.3 g) and the dosage strength (100 mg) are in different units, you must also include the equivalent relationship between these units.

100 mg = 5 mL
1,000 mg = 1 g

STEP 4: Set up the problem using equivalents as conversion factors. Start by setting up the given quantity over a denominator of 1. Make sure the units you want to cancel out appear in both the numerator and denominator.

$$\frac{0.3 \text{ g}}{1} \times \frac{1,000 \text{ mg}}{1 \text{ g}} \times \frac{5 \text{ mL}}{100 \text{ mg}}$$

STEP 5: Cancel the units that appear in both the numerator and the denominator to determine the unit of x.

$$\frac{0.3}{1} \times \frac{1,000}{1} \times \frac{5 \text{ mL}}{100}$$

STEP 6: Multiply the numerators, multiply the denominators, and divide the product of the numerators by the product of the denominators to find the answer.

$0.3 \times 1,000 \times 5 = \underline{1,500}$ (multiply the numerators)
$1 \times 1 \times 100 = \overline{100}$ (multiply the denominators)
15 (divide the products)

Administer 15 mL.

CHAPTER QUIZ

1. Order: Acetaminophen elixir 180 mg PO stat
   Available: Acetaminophen elixir 120 mg/5 mL
   How much should be administered?

   (A) 6 mL   (C) 7.2 mL

   (B) 6.5 mL   (D) 7.5 mL

2. Order: Cephalexin oral suspension 150 mg PO BID
   Available: Cephalexin oral suspension 125 mg/5 mL
   How much should be administered?

   (A) 4 mL   (C) 6 mL

   (B) 5 mL   (D) 7 mL

3. Order: Alprazolam 0.75 mg PO at bedtime
   Available: Alprazolam 0.25 mg tablets
   How much should be administered?

   (A) 2 tablets   (C) 4 tablets

   (B) 3 tablets   (D) 5 tablets

4. Order: Digoxin 0.125 mg PO daily
   Available: Digoxin 0.25 mg scored tablet
   How much should be administered?

   (A) $\frac{1}{4}$ tablet   (C) $\frac{3}{4}$ tablet

   (B) $\frac{1}{2}$ tablet   (D) 1 tablet

5. Order: Aspirin 650 mg PO TID
   Available: Aspirin 325 mg scored tablets
   How much should be administered?

   (A) 2 tablets   (C) 3 tablets

   (B) $2\frac{1}{2}$ tablets   (D) $3\frac{1}{2}$ tablets

6. Order: Furosemide oral solution 80 mg PO stat
   Available: Furosemide oral solution 10 mg/mL
   How much should be administered?

   (A) 0.8 mL   (C) 8 mL

   (B) 4.5 mL   (D) 10 mL

7. Order: Potassium chloride elixir 10 mEq PO daily
   Available: Potassium chloride elixir 20 mEq/15 mL
   How much should be administered?

   (A) 5 mL   (C) 10 mL

   (B) 7.5 mL   (D) 12.5 mL

8. Order: Ampicillin 0.5 g PO QID
   Available: Ampicillin 250 mg capsules
   How much should be administered?

   (A) 1 capsule   (C) 2 capsules

   (B) 1.5 capsules   (D) 2.5 capsules

9. Order: Ibuprofen 0.6 g PO every 8 hours prn
   Available: Ibuprofen 600 mg tablets
   How much should be administered?

   (A) 1 tablet   (C) 2 tablets

   (B) 1.5 tablets   (D) 2.5 tablets

10. Order: Ranitidine 300 mg PO at bedtime
    Available: Ranitidine 75 mg tablets
    How much should be administered?

    (A) 1 tablets   (C) 3 tablets

    (B) 2 tablets   (D) 4 tablets

ANSWERS AND EXPLANATIONS

1. D

Order: Acetaminophen elixir 180 mg PO stat.
Available: Acetaminophen elixir 120 mg/5 mL

Ratio-proportion method

180 mg : x mL :: 120 mg : 5 mL
(extremes) 900 :: 120x (means)
$$x = 7.5$$

Formula method

$$\frac{D\ (180\ mg)}{H\ (120\ mg)} \times Q\ (5\ mL) = x$$

$$\frac{180 \times 5}{120} \text{ or } \frac{900}{120} \text{ or } 7.5\ mL = x$$

Dimensional analysis

STEP 1: Identify the given quantity in the problem.

180 mg

STEP 2: Identify the wanted quantity or answer to the problem. At this time it is unknown.

x mL

STEP 3: Identify the equivalents involved in the problem. Since the given quantity and the dosage strength are in the same units, the only equivalent needed is the one provided.

120 mg = 5 mL

STEP 4: Set up the problem using equivalents as conversion factors. Start by setting up the given quantity over a denominator of 1. Make sure the units you want to cancel out appear in both the numerator and denominator.

$$\frac{180\ mg}{1} \times \frac{5\ mL}{120\ mg}$$

STEP 5: Cancel the units that appear in both the numerator and the denominator to determine the unit of x.

$$\frac{180}{1} \times \frac{5\ mL}{120}$$

STEP 6: Multiply the numerators, multiply the denominators, and divide the product of the numerators by the product of the denominators to find the answer.

$180 \times 5 = 900$ (multiply the numerators)
$1 \times 120 = 120$ (multiply the denominators)
7.5 (divide the products)

2. C

Order: Cephalexin oral suspension 150 mg PO BID
Available: Cephalexin oral suspension 125 mg/5 mL

Ratio-proportion method

150 mg : x mL :: 125 mg : 5 mL
(extremes) 750 :: 125x (means)
$$x = 6$$

Formula method

$$\frac{D\ (150\ mg)}{H\ (125\ mg)} \times Q\ (5\ mL) = x$$

$$\frac{150 \times 5}{125} \text{ or } \frac{750}{125} \text{ or } 6\ mL = x$$

Dimensional analysis

STEP 1: Identify the given quantity in the problem.

150 mg

STEP 2: Identify the wanted quantity or answer to the problem. At this time it is unknown.

x mL

STEP 3: Identify the equivalents involved in the problem. Since the given quantity and the dosage strength are in the same units, the only equivalent needed is the one provided.

125 mg = 5 mL

STEP 4: Set up the problem using equivalents as conversion factors. Start by setting up the given quantity over a denominator of 1. Make sure the units you want to cancel out appear in both the numerator and denominator.

$$\frac{150\ mg}{1} \times \frac{5\ mL}{125\ mg}$$

STEP 5: Cancel the units that appear in both the numerator and the denominator to determine the unit of x.

$$\frac{150}{1} \times \frac{5 \text{ mL}}{125}$$

STEP 6: Multiply the numerators, multiply the denominators, and divide the product of the numerators by the product of the denominators to find the answer.

$150 \times 5 = \underline{750}$ (multiply the numerators)
$1 \times 125 = \overline{125}$ (multiply the denominators)
$\qquad\quad 6$ (divide the products)

3. B

Order: Alprazolam 0.75 mg PO at bedtime
Available: Alprazolam 0.25 mg tablets

Ratio-proportion method

0.75 mg : x tablets :: 0.25 mg : 1 tablet
(extremes) 0.75 :: 0.25x (means)
$x = 3$

Formula method

$$\frac{D \ (0.75 \text{ mg})}{H \ (0.25 \text{ mg})} \times Q \ (1 \text{ tablet}) = x$$

$$\frac{0.75 \times 1}{0.25} \quad \text{or} \quad \frac{0.75}{0.25} \quad \text{or 3 tablets} = x$$

Dimensional analysis

STEP 1: Identify the given quantity in the problem.

0.75 mg

STEP 2: Identify the wanted quantity or answer to the problem. At this time it is unknown.

x tablets

STEP 3: Identify the equivalents involved in the problem. Since the given quantity and the dosage strength are in the same units, the only equivalent needed is the one provided.

0.25 mg = 1 tablet

STEP 4: Set up the problem using equivalents as conversion factors. Start by setting up the given quantity over a denominator of 1. Make sure the units you want to cancel out appear in both the numerator and denominator.

$$\frac{0.75 \text{ mg}}{1} \times \frac{1 \text{ tablet}}{0.25 \text{ mg}}$$

STEP 5: Cancel the units that appear in both the numerator and the denominator to determine the unit of x.

$$\frac{0.75}{1} \times \frac{1 \text{ tablet}}{0.25}$$

STEP 6: Multiply the numerators, multiply the denominators, and divide the product of the numerators by the product of the denominators to find the answer.

$0.75 \times 1 = \underline{0.75}$ (multiply the numerators)
$1 \times 0.25 = \overline{0.25}$ (multiply the denominators)
$\qquad\qquad 3$ (divide the products)

4. B

(Note that it is possible to give $\frac{1}{2}$ of a tablet, since the tablet is scored.)

Order: Digoxin 0.125 mg PO daily
Available: Digoxin 0.25 mg scored tablet

Ratio-proportion method

0.125 mg : x tablets :: 0.25 mg : 1 tablet
(extremes) 0.125 :: 0.25x (means)
$x = 0.5$

Formula method

$$\frac{D \ (0.125 \text{ mg})}{H \ (0.25 \text{ mg})} \times Q \ (1 \text{ tablet}) = x$$

$$\frac{0.125 \times 1}{0.25} \quad \text{or} \quad \frac{0.125}{0.25} \quad \text{or 0.5 tablet} = x$$

Dimensional analysis

STEP 1: Identify the given quantity in the problem.

0.125 mg

STEP 2: Identify the wanted quantity or answer to the problem. At this time it is unknown.

x tablets

STEP 3: Identify the equivalents involved in the problem. Since the given quantity and the dosage strength are in the same units, the only equivalent needed is the one provided.

0.25 mg = 1 tablet

STEP 4: Set up the problem using equivalents as conversion factors. Start by setting up the given quantity over a denominator of 1. Make sure the units you want to cancel out appear in both the numerator and denominator.

$$\frac{0.125 \text{ mg}}{1} \times \frac{1 \text{ tablet}}{0.25 \text{ mg}}$$

STEP 5: Cancel the units that appear in both the numerator and the denominator to determine the unit of x.

$$\frac{0.125}{1} \times \frac{1 \text{ tablet}}{0.25}$$

STEP 6: Multiply the numerators, multiply the denominators, and divide the product of the numerators by the product of the denominators to find the answer.

$0.125 \times 1 = \underline{0.125}$ (multiply the numerators)
$1 \times 0.25 = \overline{0.25}$ (multiply the denominators)
$ 0.5$ (divide the products)

5. A

Order: Aspirin 650 mg PO TID
Available: Aspirin 325 mg scored tablets

Ratio-proportion method

650 mg : x tablets :: 325 mg : 1 tablet
(extremes) 650 :: 325x (means)
$x = 2$

Formula method

$$\frac{D \text{ (650 mg)}}{H \text{ (325 mg)}} \times Q \text{ (1 tablet)} = x$$

$$\frac{650 \times 1}{325} \text{ or } \frac{650}{325} \text{ or 2 tablets} = x$$

Dimensional analysis

STEP 1: Identify the given quantity in the problem.

650 mg

STEP 2: Identify the wanted quantity or answer to the problem. At this time it is unknown.

x tablets

STEP 3: Identify the equivalents involved in the problem. Since the given quantity and the dosage strength are in the same units, the only equivalent needed is the one provided.

325 mg = 1 tablet

STEP 4: Set up the problem using equivalents as conversion factors. Start by setting up the given quantity over a denominator of 1. Make sure the units you want to cancel out appear in both the numerator and denominator.

$$\frac{650 \text{ mg}}{1} \times \frac{1 \text{ tablet}}{325 \text{ mg}}$$

STEP 5: Cancel the units that appear in both the numerator and the denominator to determine the unit of x.

$$\frac{650}{1} \times \frac{1 \text{ tablet}}{325}$$

STEP 6: Multiply the numerators, multiply the denominators, and divide the product of the numerators by the product of the denominators to find the answer.

$650 \times 1 = \underline{650}$ (multiply the numerators)
$1 \times 325 = \overline{325}$ (multiply the denominators)
$ 2$ (divide the products)

6. C

Order: Furosemide oral solution 80 mg PO stat
Available: Furosemide oral solution 10 mg/mL

Ratio-proportion method

80 mg : x mL :: 10 mg : 1 mL
(extremes) 80 :: 10x (means)
$x = 8$

Formula method

$$\frac{D \text{ (80 mg)}}{H \text{ (10 mg)}} \times Q \text{ (1 mL)} = x$$

$$\frac{80 \times 1}{10} \text{ or } \frac{80}{10} \text{ or 8 mL} = x$$

Dimensional analysis

STEP 1: Identify the given quantity in the problem.

80 mg

STEP 2: Identify the wanted quantity or answer to the problem. At this time it is unknown.

x mL

STEP 3: Identify the equivalents involved in the problem. Since the given quantity and the dosage strength are in the same units, the only equivalent needed is the one provided.

10 mg = 1 mL

STEP 4: Set up the problem using equivalents as conversion factors. Start by setting up the given quantity over a denominator of 1. Make sure the units you want to cancel out appear in both the numerator and denominator.

$$\frac{80 \text{ mg}}{1} \times \frac{1 \text{ mL}}{10 \text{ mg}}$$

STEP 5: Cancel the units that appear in both the numerator and the denominator to determine the unit of x.

$$\frac{80}{1} \times \frac{1 \text{ mL}}{10}$$

STEP 6: Multiply the numerators, multiply the denominators, and divide the product of the numerators by the product of the denominators to find the answer.

$80 \times 1 = \underline{80}$ (multiply the numerators)
$1 \times 10 = 10$ (multiply the denominators)
8 (divide the products)

7. B

Order: Potassium chloride elixir 10 mEq PO daily
Available: Potassium chloride elixir 20 mEq/15 mL

Ratio-proportion method

10 mEq:x mL :: 20 mEq:15 mL
(extremes) 150 :: 20x (means)
$x = 7.5$

Formula method

$$\frac{D\,(10 \text{ mEq})}{H\,(20 \text{ mEq})} \times Q\,(15 \text{ mL}) = x$$

$$\frac{10 \times 15}{20} \text{ or } \frac{150}{20} \text{ or } 7.5 \text{ mL} = x$$

Dimensional analysis

STEP 1: Identify the given quantity in the problem.

10 mEq

STEP 2: Identify the wanted quantity or answer to the problem. At this time it is unknown.

x mL

STEP 3: Identify the equivalents involved in the problem. Since the given quantity and the dosage strength are in the same units, the only equivalent needed is the one provided.

20 mEq = 15 mL

STEP 4: Set up the problem using equivalents as conversion factors. Start by setting up the given quantity over a denominator of 1. Make sure the units you want to cancel out appear in both the numerator and denominator.

$$\frac{10 \text{ mEq}}{1} \times \frac{15 \text{ mL}}{20 \text{ mEq}}$$

STEP 5: Cancel the units that appear in both the numerator and the denominator to determine the unit of your answer.

$$\frac{10}{1} \times \frac{15 \text{ mL}}{20}$$

STEP 6: Multiply the numerators, multiply the denominators, and divide the product of the numerators by the product of the denominators to find the answer.

$10 \times 15 = \underline{150}$ (multiply the numerators)
$1 \times 20 = 20$ (multiply the denominators)
7.5 (divide the products)

8. C

Since it is not possible to split a capsule, options (B) and (D) are not logical answers.

Order: Ampicillin 0.5 g PO QID
Available: Ampicillin 250 mg capsules

Ratio-proportion method

Note: You must first convert 0.5 g into 500 mg.

500 mg : x capsules :: 250 mg : 1 capsule
(extremes) 500 :: 250x (means)
$$x = 2$$

Formula method

Note: You must first convert 0.5 g into 500 mg.

$$\frac{D \,(500 \text{ mg})}{H \,(250 \text{ mg})} \times Q \,(1 \text{ capsule}) = x$$

$$\frac{500 \times 1}{250} \quad \text{or} \quad \frac{500}{250} \quad \text{or 2 capsules} = x$$

Dimensional analysis

STEP 1: Identify the given quantity in the problem.

0.5 g

STEP 2: Identify the wanted quantity or answer to the problem. At this time it is unknown.

x capsules

STEP 3: Identify the equivalents involved in the problem. One equivalent relationship is provided. Since the given quantity (0.5 g) and the dosage strength (250 mg) are in different units, you must also include the equivalent relationship between these units.

250 mg = 1 capsule
1,000 mg = 1 g

STEP 4: Set up the problem using equivalents as conversion factors. Start by setting up the given quantity over a denominator of 1. Make sure the units you want to cancel out appear in both the numerator and denominator.

$$\frac{0.5 \text{ g}}{1} \times \frac{1,000 \text{ mg}}{1 \text{ g}} \times \frac{1 \text{ capsule}}{250 \text{ mg}}$$

STEP 5: Cancel the units that appear in both the numerator and the denominator to determine the unit of x.

$$\frac{0.5}{1} \times \frac{1,000}{1} \times \frac{1 \text{ capsule}}{250}$$

STEP 6: Multiply the numerators, multiply the denominators, and divide the product of the numerators by the product of the denominators to find the answer.

$0.5 \times 1,000 \times 1 = \underline{500}$ (multiply the numerators)
$1 \times 1 \times 250 = \overline{250}$ (multiply the denominators)
2 (divide the products)

9. A

Order: Ibuprofen 0.6 g PO every 8 hours prn
Available: Ibuprofen 600 mg tablets

Ratio-proportion method

Note: You must first convert 0.6 g into 600 mg.

600 mg : x tablets :: 600 mg : 1 tablet
(extremes) 600 :: 600x (means)
$$x = 1$$

Note: After converting 0.6 g into 600 mg, it should not be necessary to continue with the calculation, as the answer would be obvious.

Formula method

Note: You must first convert 0.6 g into 600 mg.

$$\frac{D \,(600 \text{ mg})}{H \,(600 \text{ mg})} \times Q \,(1 \text{ tablet}) = x$$

$$\frac{600 \times 1}{600} \quad \text{or} \quad \frac{600}{600} \quad \text{or 1 tablet} = x$$

Dimensional analysis

STEP 1: Identify the given quantity in the problem.

0.6 g

STEP 2: Identify the wanted quantity or answer to the problem. At this time it is unknown.

x tablets

STEP 3: Identify the equivalents involved in the problem. One equivalent relationship is provided. Since the given quantity (0.6 g) and the dosage strength (600 mg) are in different units, you must also include the equivalent relationship between these units.

600 mg = 1 tablet
1,000 mg = 1 g

STEP 4: Set up the problem using equivalents as conversion factors. Start by setting up the given quantity over a denominator of 1. Make sure the units you want to cancel out appear in both the numerator and denominator.

$$\frac{0.6\ g}{1} \times \frac{1,000\ mg}{1\ g} \times \frac{1\ tablet}{600\ mg}$$

STEP 5: Cancel the units that appear in both the numerator and the denominator to determine the unit of x.

$$\frac{0.6}{1} \times \frac{1,000}{1} \times \frac{1\ tablet}{600}$$

STEP 6: Multiply the numerators, multiply the denominators, and divide the product of the numerators by the product of the denominators to find the answer.

$0.6 \times 1,000 \times 1 = \underline{600}$ (multiply the numerators)
$1 \times 1 \times 600 = \overline{600}$ (multiply the denominators)
$\qquad\qquad\qquad 1$ (divide the products)

10. D

Order: Ranitidine 300 mg PO at bedtime
Available: Ranitidine 75 mg tablets

Ratio-proportion method

300 mg : x tablets :: 75 mg : 1 tablet
(extremes) 300 :: 75x (means)
$\qquad\qquad x = 4$

Formula method

$$\frac{D\ (300\ mg)}{H\ (75\ mg)} \times Q\ (1\ tablet) = x$$

$\frac{300 \times 1}{75}$ or $\frac{300}{75}$ or 4 tablets $= x$

Dimensional analysis

STEP 1: Identify the given quantity in the problem.

300 mg

STEP 2: Identify the wanted quantity or answer to the problem. At this time it is unknown.

x tablets

STEP 3: Identify the equivalents involved in the problem. Since the given quantity and the dosage strength are in the same units, the only equivalent needed is the one provided.

75 mg = 1 tablet

STEP 4: Set up the problem using equivalents as conversion factors. Start by setting up the given quantity over a denominator of 1. Make sure the units you want to cancel out appear in both the numerator and denominator.

$$\frac{300\ mg}{1} \times \frac{1\ tablet}{75\ mg}$$

STEP 5: Cancel the units that appear in both the numerator and the denominator to determine the unit of x.

$$\frac{300}{1} \times \frac{1\ tablet}{75}$$

STEP 6: Multiply the numerators, multiply the denominators, and divide the product of the numerators by the product of the denominators to find the answer.

$300 \times 1 = \underline{300}$ (multiply the numerators)
$1 \times 75 = \overline{75}$ (multiply the denominators)
$\qquad\qquad 4$ (divide the products)

CHAPTER 10

Parenteral Medications

Parenteral medication refers to any medication that is not given through the gastrointestinal tract. These medication routes include intramuscular, subcutaneous, and intravenous. Because these medications cannot be recalled once administered, it is imperative that their doses be accurately calculated. This chapter will discuss solving intramuscular and subcutaneous medication problems using four different methods: the ratio-proportion method (two formats), the formula method, and dimensional analysis.

CALCULATING PARENTERAL MEDICATION ADMINISTRATION VOLUMES

When calculating dosages for parenteral medications, be sure to review the rounding guidelines for each specific care area. Generally, volumes less than 1 mL are rounded to the hundredths place, and volumes greater than 1 mL are rounded to the tenths place. Consider the following raw answers and their corresponding rounded answers:

Raw answer	Rounding convention	Rounded answer
0.235	Rounded to nearest hundredth:	0.24
0.922	Rounded to nearest hundredth:	0.92
1.347	Rounded to nearest tenth:	1.3
3.75	Rounded to nearest tenth:	3.8
0.95	Rounded to nearest hundredth:	0.95 (unchanged; already calculated to nearest hundredth)

0.5 mL and 1 mL syringes are used for administering intramuscular and subcutaneous medications. Occasionally an injection will exceed 1 mL, in which case a 2 mL syringe would be appropriate. Syringes intended for injections are often graduated in 0.1 mL or even 0.01 mL increments. Always use the smallest syringe that will hold the entire amount of medication in order to enhance accuracy when drawing up the medication. For example, when administering a volume of 0.75 mL, choose a 1 mL syringe; for a volume of 0.25 mL, choose a 0.5 mL syringe.

Let's solve the following parenteral medication problems using each method.

Example 1:

> Physician-ordered dose: Azactam 750 mg IM every 8 hours
> Dose available: Azactam 1 g/5 mL vial

First, look at the doses. To be solved correctly, the weight of the doses must use the same units of measurement. If the dose weights are in different units of measurement, make a conversion to the same unit. In this problem, are the medication ordered and the available form in the same units? No, they are not. Therefore, a unit conversion must be made.

> **Math Tip:** It is usually a good idea to convert to the smaller unit of measurement. This decreases the chance of misplacing a decimal point.

Ratio-proportion methods

Make any necessary conversions: 1 g = 1,000 mg.

Set up using either the means:extremes format or the fraction format.

Means:extremes format:

$$extremes : means = means : extremes$$

Now enter the values for this problem.

(number of mg/mL available) 1,000 mg : 5 mL = 750 mg : x mL (ordered mg/unknown mL)
(multiply the means) 3,750 = 1,000x (multiply the extremes)
(divide both sides by 1,000) 3,750 ÷ 1,000 = 1,000x ÷ 1,000
$$3.75 = x$$

Since the dose is greater than 1 mL, round to the tenth; 3.8 mL should be given to the patient.

Fraction format:

Make any necessary conversions: 1 g = 1,000 mg.

Set up the problem in fraction form.

$$\frac{\text{available mL}}{\text{available mg}} \diagdown\!\!\!= \frac{\text{unknown mL}}{\text{ordered mg}}$$

$$\frac{5 \text{ mL}}{1,000 \text{ mg}} = \frac{x}{750 \text{ mg}}$$

Cross multiply and solve for x.

$$1{,}000x = 3{,}750$$
$$x = 3.75 \text{ mL}$$

Since the dose is greater than 1 mL, round to the tenth; 3.8 mL should be given to the patient.

Formula method

Make any necessary conversions: 1 g = 1,000 mg.

Set up the problem using the following formula.

$$\frac{D}{H} \times Q$$

D is the "desired" or ordered dose.

H is the "have" or amount available.

Q is the "quantity" or the volume the "have" is found in.

$$\text{desired} \rightarrow \underset{\text{have} \rightarrow 1{,}000 \text{ mg}}{\frac{750 \text{ mg}}{}} \times 5 \text{ mL} \leftarrow \text{quantity}$$

Divide: $750 \div 1{,}000 = 0.75$

Multiply: $0.75 \times 5 \text{ mL} = 3.75 \text{ mL}$

Since this answer is greater than 1 mL, round to the tenth; the patient should be given 3.8 mL.

Dimensional analysis

Make any necessary unit conversions: 1 g = 1,000 mg.

Identify the desired quantity and set it over a denominator of 1. Identify the equivalents given in the problem (1,000 mg per 5 mL) and set them up as a conversion factor. Make sure any duplicate units appear in both the numerator and denominator.

$$x = \underset{\text{1 (constant)}}{\overset{\text{(ordered dose)}}{\frac{\text{Desired}}{}}} \times \underset{\text{Equivalent (unit same as Desired)}}{\overset{\text{(available dose)}}{\frac{\text{Equivalent (unit different from Desired)}}{}}}$$

Cancel out the units that appear in both the numerator and denominator, and multiply straight across.

$$x = \frac{750}{1} \times \frac{5 \text{ mL}}{1{,}000} = \frac{3{,}750}{1{,}000} \quad \begin{array}{l} \text{(multiply the numerators)} \\ \text{(multiply the denominators)} \end{array}$$

Divide the products: $3{,}750 \div 1{,}000 = 3.75$.

Round to the nearest tenth: $x = 3.8 \text{ mL}$.

The patient should receive 3.8 mL.

Example 2:

> Physician-ordered dose: Estradiol valerate 30 mg IM weekly
> Dose available: Estradiol valerate 40 mg/mL

Ratio-proportion methods

Set up using either the means:extremes format or fraction format for the ratio-proportion method.

The means:extremes method is set up in the following manner:

$$\text{extremes:means} = \text{means:extremes}$$

Means:extremes format:

No conversions are necessary for this problem.

> (number of mg/mL available) 40 mg:1 mL = 30 mg:x mL (ordered mg/unknown mL)
> (multiply the means) 30 = 40x (multiply the extremes)
> (divide both sides by 40) 30 ÷ 40 = 40x ÷ 40
> 0.75 = x

Any dose less than 1 mL should be rounded to the hundredth. This answer is already stated to the hundredth, so no rounding is needed; 0.75 mL should be administered to the patient.

Fraction format:

No conversions are necessary for this problem.

Set up the problem in fraction form.

$$\frac{\text{available mL}}{\text{available mg}} = \frac{\text{unknown mL}}{\text{ordered mg}}$$

Now enter the values for this problem.

$$\frac{1 \text{ mL}}{40 \text{ mg}} \diagup\!\!\!\!\!= \frac{x}{30 \text{ mg}}$$

Cross multiply and solve for x.

> 40x = 30
> x = 0.75 mL

Since this dose is less than 1 mL and already stated to the hundredth, no rounding is needed; 0.75 mL should be given to the patient.

Formula method

$$\frac{D}{H} \times Q$$

No conversions are necessary for this problem.

$$\text{desired} \rightarrow \frac{30 \text{ mg}}{40 \text{ mg}} \leftarrow \text{have} \times 1 \text{ mL} \leftarrow \text{quantity}$$

Divide: $30 \div 40 = 0.75$

Multiply: $0.75 \times 1 \text{ mL} = 0.75 \text{ mL}$

Since this dose is less than 1 mL and already stated to the hundredth, no rounding is needed. The patient should be given 0.75 mL.

Dimensional analysis

No conversions are necessary for this problem.

$$x = \frac{\overset{\text{(ordered dose)}}{\text{Desired}}}{1 \text{ (constant)}} \times \frac{\overset{\text{(available dose)}}{\text{Equivalent (unit different from Desired)}}}{\text{Equivalent (unit same as Desired)}}$$

$$x = \frac{30 \text{ mg}}{1} \times \frac{1 \text{ mL}}{40 \text{ mg}}$$

$$x = \frac{30}{1} \times \frac{1 \text{ mL}}{40} = \begin{matrix} 30 \\ 40 \end{matrix} \quad \begin{matrix} \text{(multiply the numerators)} \\ \text{(multiply the denominators)} \end{matrix}$$

Divide the products: $30 \div 40 = 0.75$.

No rounding is needed. The patient should receive 0.75 mL.

Practice 1

Solve the following problems for practice, using your method of choice. Round answers less than 1 mL to the hundredth and answers greater than 1 mL to the tenth.

1. Physician-ordered dose: Bactocill 250 mg IM every 6 hours
    Dose available: Bactocill 1 g/3 mL

2. Physician-ordered dose: Robaxin 225 mg IM every 8 hours prn
    Dose available: Robaxin 100 mg/mL

RECONSTITUTION AND CALCULATION OF PARENTERAL MEDICATIONS

Many medications are unstable in liquid form and, therefore, are dispensed from the pharmacy in powdered form. For these medications, the nurse will have to reconstitute the medication prior to administering it to the patient. The following examples outline how to solve these problems.

> **Math Tip:** The action of reconstituting the medication to the proper strength is important but not for this type of drug calculation. Once the drug is reconstituted, the amount used to reconstitute is considered unnecessary information. After you disregard this information, set up this type of dosage calculation problem using your method of choice and solve as you did for the previous dosage calculations.

Example 1:

Physician-ordered dose: Ticar 500 mg IM

Dose available: Directions on label. Add 2 mL sterile water to make Ticar 1 g/2.6 mL.

Make all necessary conversions prior to setting up any equation. For this problem, convert 1 g to 1,000 mg.

Disregard the information regarding the volume needed for reconstitution; it is unnecessary for this type of drug calculation.

Round all answers less than 1 mL to the hundredth and answers greater than 1 mL to the tenth.

Ratio-proportion methods

Means : extremes format:

$$\text{extremes : means} = \text{means : extremes}$$

(number of mg/mL available) 1,000 mg : 2.6 mL = 500 mg : x mL (ordered mg/unknown mL)

(multiply the means) 1,300 = 1,000x (multiply the extremes)

(divide both sides by 1,000) 1,300 ÷ 1,000 = 1,000x ÷ 1,000

$$1.3 = x$$

No rounding is needed. The patient should be given 1.3 mL.

Fraction format:

Set up the problem in fraction form.

$$\frac{\text{available mL}}{\text{available mg}} = \frac{\text{unknown mL}}{\text{ordered mg}}$$

Now enter the values for this problem.

$$\frac{2.6\ \text{mL}}{1,000\ \text{mg}} \diagdown\!\!\!\!\diagup \frac{x}{500\ \text{mg}}$$

Cross multiply and solve for *x*.

$$1,000x = 1,300$$
$$x = 1.3$$

No rounding is needed; the patient should be given 1.3 mL.

Formula method

$$\begin{array}{l}\text{desired} \rightarrow \\ \text{have} \rightarrow\end{array} \frac{500\ \text{mg}}{1,000\ \text{mg}} \times 2.6\ \text{mL} \leftarrow \text{quantity}$$

Divide: 500 ÷ 1,000 = 0.5

Multiply: 0.5 × 2.6 mL = 1.3 mL

Dimensional analysis

$$x = \frac{500 \text{ mg}}{1} \times \frac{2.6 \text{ mL}}{1{,}000 \text{ mg}}$$

Cancel out the units that appear in both the numerator and denominator, and multiply straight across.

$$x = \frac{500}{1} \times \frac{2.6 \text{ mL}}{1{,}000} = \frac{1{,}300}{1{,}000} \quad \begin{array}{l} \text{(multiply the numerators)} \\ \text{(multiply the denominators)} \end{array}$$

Divide the products: 1,300 mL ÷ 1,000 = 1.3 mL.

No rounding is needed; the patient should be given 1.3 mL.

Example 2:

> Physician-ordered dose: Cefazolin sodium 0.5 g every 6 hours
> Dose available: Add 2.5 mL sterile water for injection to make cefazolin sodium 330 mg/mL.

Make all necessary conversions prior to setting up any equations. For this problem, convert 0.5 g to 500 mg.

Disregard the information regarding the volume need for reconstitution; it is unnecessary information for this type of drug calculation.

Ratio-proportion methods

Means : extremes format:

$$\text{extremes} : \text{means} = \text{means} : \text{extremes}$$

(number of mg/mL available) 330 mg : 1 mL = 500 mg : x mL (ordered mg/unknown mL)
(multiply the means) 500 = 330x (multiply the extremes)
(divide both sides by 330) 550 ÷ 330 = 330x ÷ 330
$$1.515\ldots = x$$

Round to the nearest tenth; the patient should be given 1.5 mL.

Fraction format:

$$\frac{1 \text{ mL}}{330 \text{ mg}} \diagdown\!\!\!\!\diagup \frac{x}{500 \text{ mg}}$$

Cross multiply and solve for x.

$$330x = 500$$
$$x = 1.515\ldots$$

Round to a final answer of 1.5 mL.

Formula method

$$\text{desired} \rightarrow \frac{500 \text{ mg}}{330 \text{ mg}} \times 1 \text{ mL} \leftarrow \text{quantity}$$
$$\text{have} \rightarrow$$

Divide: $500 \div 330 = 1.515\ldots$

Multiply: $1.515\ldots \times 1 \text{ mL} = 1.515\ldots \text{ mL}$

Round to a final answer of 1.5 mL.

Dimensional analysis

$$x = \frac{500 \text{ mg}}{1} \times \frac{1 \text{ mL}}{330 \text{ mg}}$$

Cancel out the units that appear in both the numerator and denominator, and multiply straight across.

$$x = \frac{500}{1} \times \frac{1 \text{ mL}}{330} = \frac{500}{330} \quad \begin{array}{l} \text{(multiply the numerators)} \\ \text{(multiply the denominators)} \end{array}$$

Divide the products: $500 \text{ mL} \div 330 = 1.515\ldots \text{ mL}$

Round to a final answer of 1.5 mL.

Practice 2

Using your method of choice, solve the following problems. Round volumes less than 1 mL to the hundredth and volumes greater than 1 mL to the tenth.

1. Physician-ordered dose: Penicillin G 300,000 units IM

   Dose available and reconstitution directions:
   Add 9.6 mL NS to make penicillin G 100,000 units/mL.

2. Physician-ordered dose: Cefadyl 700 mg IM

   Dose available and reconstitution directions:
   Add 1 mL NS to make cefadyl 500 mg/1.2 mL.

ADMINISTRATION OF DRUGS AVAILABLE IN UNITS

Some drugs, such as insulin and heparin, are dosed in units rather than milligrams. Heparin often comes as 5,000 units per 1 mL and can be dosed using a standard 1 mL syringe. Insulin, on the other hand, is *always* dosed using an insulin syringe. The standard concentration for all insulins is 100 units per mL; this concentration is referred to as U-100. Insulin syringes are graduated (that is, marked) in terms of units rather than volume. To administer 12 units of insulin, for example, the nurse would select a vial of U-100 insulin and a matching U-100 syringe. Occasionally a more concentrated form of insulin is called for. For example, insulin may be packaged as U-500, which contains 500 units per mL. When administering U-500 insulin, the nurse must use a U-500 syringe.

ANSWERS AND EXPLANATIONS TO PRACTICE EXERCISES

Practice 1

1. 0.75 mL

Make any necessary conversions for this problem:

1 g = 1,000 mg (use this conversion for all methods).

Ratio-proportion methods

Means : extremes format:

(number of mg/mL available) 1,000 mg : 3 mL = 250 mg : x mL (ordered mg/unknown mL)

(multiply the means) 1,000 = 750x (multiply the extremes)

(divide both sides by 750) 1,000 ÷ 750 = 750x ÷ 750

$$0.75 = x$$

The result, 0.75 mL, is less than 1 mL and is already expressed in hundredths, so no rounding is needed. The patient should be given 0.75 mL.

Fraction format:

$$\frac{3\text{ mL}}{1,000\text{ mg}} \diagdown\!\!\!\!\diagup \frac{x}{250\text{ mg}}$$

Cross multiply and find x.

$$1,000x = 750$$
$$x = 0.75\text{ mL}$$

No rounding is needed; the patient should be given 0.75 mL.

Formula method

$$\text{desired} \rightarrow \frac{250\text{ mg}}{1,000\text{ mg}} \leftarrow \text{have} \times 3\text{ mL} \leftarrow \text{quantity}$$

Divide: 250 ÷ 1,000 = 0.25

Multiply: 0.25 × 3 mL = 0.75 mL

No rounding is needed; the patient should be given 0.75 mL.

Dimensional analysis

$$x = \frac{250\text{ mg}}{1} \times \frac{3\text{ mL}}{1,000\text{ mg}}$$

Cancel out the units that appear in both the numerator and denominator, and multiply straight across.

$$x = \frac{250}{1} \times \frac{3\text{ mL}}{1,000} = \frac{750}{1,000}\quad\begin{array}{l}\text{(multiply the numerators)}\\\text{(multiply the denominators)}\end{array}$$

Divide the products: 750 mL ÷ 1,000 = 0.75 mL.

No rounding is needed; the patient should be given 0.75 mL.

2. 2.3 mL

No conversions are necessary for this problem.

Ratio-proportion methods

Means : extremes format:

(number of mg/mL available) 100 mg : 1 mL = 225 mg : x mL (ordered mg/unknown mL)
(multiply the means) $225 = 100x$ (multiply the extremes)
(divide both sides by 100) $225 \div 100 = 100x \div 100$
$$2.25 = x$$

Since the volume is greater than 1, round to the nearest tenth for a final answer of 2.3 mL.

Fraction format:

$$\frac{1 \text{ mL}}{100 \text{ mg}} \times \frac{x}{225 \text{ mg}}$$

Cross multiply and solve for x.

$$100x = 225$$
$$x = 2.25 \text{ mL}$$

Round to the nearest tenth for a final answer of 2.3 mL.

Formula method

$$\frac{\text{desired} \rightarrow 225 \text{ mg}}{\text{have} \rightarrow 100 \text{ mg}} \times 1 \text{ mL} \leftarrow \text{quantity}$$

Divide: $225 \div 100 = 2.25$

Multiply: $2.25 \times 1 \text{ mL} = 2.25 \text{ mL}$

Round the final answer to 2.3 mL.

Dimensional analysis

$$x = \frac{225 \text{ mg}}{1} \times \frac{1 \text{ mL}}{100 \text{ mg}}$$

Cancel out the units that appear in both the numerator and denominator, and multiply straight across.

$$x = \frac{225}{1} \times \frac{1 \text{ mL}}{100} = \frac{250}{100} \quad \begin{array}{l}\text{(multiply the numerators)}\\\text{(multiply the denominators)}\end{array}$$

Divide the products: $225 \text{ mL} \div 100 = 2.25 \text{ mL}$.

Round 2.25 to the nearest tenth to get 2.3 mL.

Practice 2

1. 3 mL

No conversions are necessary for this problem.

Ratio-proportion methods

Means:extremes format:

(number of units/mL available) 100,000 units:1 = 300,000 units:x mL (ordered units/unknown mL)

(multiply the means) 300,000 = 100,000x (multiply the extremes)

(divide both sides by 100,000) 300,000 ÷ 100,000 = 100,000x ÷ 100,000

$$3 = x$$

The patient should be given 3 mL.

Fraction format:

$$\frac{1 \text{ mL}}{100,000 \text{ units}} \times \frac{x}{300,000 \text{ units}}$$

Cross multiply and solve for x.

$$100,000x = 300,000$$
$$x = 3$$

The patient should be given 3 mL.

Formula method

$$\begin{array}{l}\text{desired} \rightarrow \\ \text{have} \rightarrow\end{array} \frac{300,000 \text{ mg}}{100,000 \text{ mg}} \times 1 \text{ mL} \leftarrow \text{quantity}$$

Divide: 300,000 ÷ 100,000 = 3

Multiply: 3 × 1 mL = 3 mL

The patient should be given 3 mL.

Dimensional analysis

$$x = \frac{300,000 \text{ units}}{1} \times \frac{1 \text{ mL}}{100,000 \text{ mg}}$$

Cancel out the units that appear in both the numerator and denominator, and multiply straight across.

$$x = \frac{300,000}{1} \times \frac{1 \text{ mL}}{100,000} = \frac{300,000}{100,000} \quad \begin{array}{l}\text{(multiply the numerators)}\\\text{(multiply the denominators)}\end{array}$$

Divide the products: 300,000 mL ÷ 100,000 = 3 mL.

The patient should be given 3 mL.

2. 1.7 mL

Ratio-proportion methods

No conversions are necessary for this problem.

Means : extremes format:

(number of mg/mL available) 500 mg : 1.2 mL = 700 mg : x mL (ordered mg/unknown mL)

(multiply the means) 840 = 500x (multiply the extremes)

(divide both sides by 500) 840 ÷ 500 = 500x ÷ 500

$$1.68 = x$$

Round 1.68 to the nearest tenth; the patient should be given 1.7 mL.

Fraction format:

$$\frac{1.2 \text{ mL}}{500 \text{ mg}} \diagup\!\!\!\!= \frac{x}{700 \text{ mg}}$$

Cross multiply and solve for x.

$$500x = 840$$
$$x = 1.68$$

Round 1.68 to the nearest tenth; the patient should be given 1.7 mL.

Formula method

$$\begin{array}{c}\text{desired} \rightarrow \\ \text{have} \rightarrow\end{array} \frac{700 \text{ mg}}{500 \text{ mg}} \times 1.2 \text{ mL} \leftarrow \text{quantity}$$

Divide: 700 ÷ 500 = 1.4

Multiply: 1.4 × 1.2 mL = 1.68 mL

Round 1.68 to the nearest tenth; the patient should be given 1.7 mL.

Dimensional analysis

$$x = \frac{700 \text{ mg}}{1} \times \frac{1.2 \text{ mL}}{500 \text{ mg}}$$

Cancel out the units that appear in both the numerator and denominator, and multiply straight across.

$$x = \frac{700}{1} \times \frac{1.2 \text{ mL}}{500} \begin{array}{l} = 840 \quad \text{(multiply the numerators)} \\ = 500 \quad \text{(multiply the denominators)}\end{array}$$

Divide the products: 840 mL ÷ 500 = 1.68 mL.

Round 1.68 to the nearest tenth; the patient should be given 1.7 mL.

CHAPTER QUIZ

Using your method of choice, solve the following parenteral medication problems. All three methods (and relevant alternative formats) are included in the chapter quiz answers and explanations. Round doses greater than 1 mL to the tenth and doses less than 1 mL to the hundredth.

1. Physician-ordered dose: Meperidine 75 mg
   IM q 4 hr prn

   Dose available: Meperidine 40 mg/mL

   (A) 0.53 mL   (C) 1.9 mL

   (B) 1.87 mL   (D) 2.5 mL

2. Physician-ordered dose: Atropine sulfate
   0.4 mg IM

   Dose available: Atropine sulfate
   0.6 mg/mL

   (A) .67 mL   (C) 0.67 mL

   (B) .66 mL   (D) 0.66 mL

3. Physician-ordered dose: Potassium chloride
   25 mEq IVPB

   Dose available: Potassium chloride
   40 mEq/10 mL

   How much should be added to the IVPB
   solution?

   (A) 1.6 mL   (C) 100 mL

   (B) 6.25 mL   (D) 6.3 mL

4. Physician-ordered dose: Kanamycin 200 mg IM

   Dose available and reconstitution directions:
   Add 2.3 mL sterile water to make kanamycin
   1 g/3 mL.

   (A) 0.66 mL   (C) 0.6 mL

   (B) 0.4 mL   (D) .46 mL

5. Physician-ordered dose: Benadryl 75 mg
   IVP STAT

   Dose available: Benadryl 50 mg/mL

   (A) 1.2 mL   (C) 1.3 mL

   (B) 1.5 mL   (D) 1.4 mL

6. Physician-ordered dose: Dilantin 100 mg IVP

   Dose available: Dilantin 50 mg/mL

   (A) 0.5 mL   (C) 1.9 mL
   (B) 2 mL   (D) 2.2 mL

7. Physician-ordered dose: Chlorpromazine
   Hydrochloride 40 mg IM q 6 hr prn

   Dose available: Chlorpromazine hydrochloride
   25 mg/mL

   (A) 1.6 mL   (C) 0.6 mL
   (B) 1.60 mL   (D) 1.3 mL

8. Physician-ordered dose: Heparin 800 units
   sub-q bid

   Dose available: Heparin 5,000 units/mL

   (A) 0.2 mL   (C) 1.6 mL
   (B) 0.12 mL   (D) 0.16 mL

9. Physician-ordered dose: Ticar 1,000 mg IM q 6 hours

   Dose available and reconstitution instructions: Add 2 mL sterile water for injection to make 1 g/2.6 mL.

   (A) 2 mL   (C) 2.6 mL

   (B) 0.8 mL   (D) 1.8 mL

10. Physician-ordered dose: Piperacillin sodium 1,875 mg IM every 4 hours

   Dose available: Reconstitute with 2 mL of sterile water to make piperacillin sodium 1 g/2.5 mL.

   (A) 4.68 mL   (C) 3.8 mL

   (B) 3.75 mL   (D) 4.7 mL

ANSWERS AND EXPLANATIONS

1. C

No conversions are necessary for this problem.

Ratio-proportion methods

Means : extremes format:

(number of mg/mL available) 40 mg : 1 mL = 75 mg : x mL (ordered mg/unknown mL)

(multiply the means) 75 = 40x (multiply the extremes)

(divide both sides by 40) 75 ÷ 40 = 40x ÷ 40

1.875 = x

Round 1.875 to the nearest tenth for a final answer of 1.9 mL.

Fraction format:

Set up the problem in fraction form.

$$\frac{\text{available mL}}{\text{available mg}} = \frac{\text{unknown mL}}{\text{ordered mg}}$$

Now enter the values for this problem.

$$\frac{1 \text{ mL}}{40 \text{ mg}} \diagdown\!\!\!\!= \frac{x}{75 \text{ mg}}$$

Cross multiply and find x.

40x = 75

x = 1.875

Round to the nearest tenth: 1.9 mL.

Formula method

$$\begin{array}{l}\text{desired} \rightarrow \\ \text{have} \rightarrow\end{array} \frac{75 \text{ mg}}{40 \text{ mg}} \times 1 \text{ mL} \leftarrow \text{quantity}$$

Divide: 75 ÷ 40 = 1.875

Multiply: 1.875 × 1 mL = 1.875 mL

Round 1.875 to the nearest tenth for a final answer of 1.9 mL.

Dimensional analysis

$$x = \frac{\overset{\text{(ordered dose)}}{\text{Desired}}}{1 \text{ (constant)}} \times \frac{\overset{\text{(available dose)}}{\text{Equivalent (unit different from Desired)}}}{\text{Equivalent (unit same as Desired)}}$$

$$x = \frac{75 \text{ ml}}{1} \times \frac{1 \text{ mL}}{40 \text{ mg}}$$

Cancel out the units that appear in both the numerator and denominator, and multiply straight across.

$$x = \frac{75}{1} \times \frac{1 \text{ mL}}{40} = \begin{array}{l} 75 \text{ (multiply the numerators)} \\ 40 \text{ (multiply the denominators)} \end{array}$$

Divide the products: 75 mL ÷ 40 = 1.875 mL.

Round to 1.9 mL.

2. C

No conversions are necessary for this problem.

Ratio-proportion methods

Means : extremes format:

(number of mg/mL available) 0.6 mg : 1 mL = 0.4 mg : x mL (ordered mg/unknown mL)

(multiply the means) 0.4 = 0.6x (multiply the extremes)

(divide both sides by 0.6) 0.4x ÷ 0.6 = 0.6x ÷ 0.6

0.666... = x

Round 0.666... to the nearest hundredth for a final answer of 0.67 mL.

Fraction format:

$$\frac{1\ mL}{0.6\ mg} \diagdown\mkern-18mu\diagup\mkern-6mu= \frac{x}{0.4\ mg}$$

Cross multiply and solve for x.

0.6x = 0.4

x = 0.666...

Round 0.666... to the nearest hundredth: 0.67 mL.

Formula method

$$\text{desired} \rightarrow \frac{0.4\ mg}{0.6\ mg} \leftarrow \text{have} \times 1\ mL \leftarrow \text{quantity}$$

Divide: 0.4 ÷ 0.6 = 0.666...

Multiply: 0.666... × 1 mL = 0.666... mL

Round to the nearest hundredth: 0.67 mL.

Dimensional analysis

$$x = \frac{0.4\ mg}{1} \times \frac{1\ mL}{0.6\ mg}$$

Cancel out the units that appear in both the numerator and denominator, and multiply straight across.

$$x = \frac{0.4}{1} \times \frac{1\ mL}{0.6} = \frac{0.4}{0.6} \quad \begin{array}{l}\text{(multiply the numerators)}\\ \text{(multiply the denominators)}\end{array}$$

Divide the products: 0.4 mL ÷ 0.6 = 0.666...

Round 1.666... to the nearest hundredth: 0.67 mL.

3. D

No conversions are necessary for this problem.

Ratio-proportion methods

Means : extremes format:

(number of mEq/mL available) 40 mEq : 10 mL = 25 mEq : x mL (ordered mEq/unknown mL)

(multiply the means) 250 = 40x (multiply the extremes)

(divide both sides by 40) 250 ÷ 40 = 40x ÷ 40

$$6.25 = x$$

Round 6.25 to the nearest tenth for a final answer of 6.3 mL.

Fraction format:

$$\frac{10 \text{ mL}}{40 \text{ mEq}} \times \frac{x}{25 \text{ mEq}}$$

Cross multiply and solve for x.

$$40x = 250$$
$$x = 6.25$$

Round 6.25 to the nearest tenth: 6.3 mL.

Formula method

$$\begin{array}{c}\text{desired} \rightarrow \\ \text{have} \rightarrow\end{array} \frac{25 \text{ mEq}}{40 \text{ mEq}} \times 10 \text{ mL} \leftarrow \text{quantity}$$

Divide: 25 ÷ 40 = 0.625

Multiply: 0.625 × 10 mL = 6.25 mL

Round 6.25 to the nearest tenth: 6.3 mL.

Dimensional analysis

$$x = \frac{25 \text{ mEq}}{1} \times \frac{10 \text{ mL}}{40 \text{ mEq}}$$

Cancel out the units that appear in both the numerator and denominator, and multiply straight across.

$$x = \frac{25}{1} \times \frac{10 \text{ mL}}{40} = \frac{250}{40} \quad \begin{array}{l}\text{(multiply the numerators)} \\ \text{(multiply the denominators)}\end{array}$$

Divide the products: 250 mL ÷ 40 = 6.25 mL.

Round 6.25 to the nearest tenth: 6.3 mL.

4. C

Convert 1 g to 1,000 mg (use this conversion for all methods). Disregard the information regarding the volume needed for reconstitution; it is unnecessary for this type of drug calculation.

Ratio-proportion methods

Means : extremes format:

(number of mg/mL available) 1,000 mg : 3 mL = 200 mg : x mL (ordered mg/unknown mL)
(multiply the means) 600 = 1,000x (multiply the extremes)
(divide both sides by 1,000) 600 ÷ 1,000 = 1,000x ÷ 1,000
0.6 = x

No rounding is needed. The patient should be given 0.6 mL.

Fraction format:

$$\frac{1 \text{ mL}}{1,000 \text{ mg}} = \frac{x}{600 \text{ mg}}$$

Cross multiply and solve for x.

$$1,000x = 600$$
$$x = 0.6$$

No rounding is needed. The patient should be given 0.6 mL.

Formula method

$$\frac{\text{desired} \rightarrow\ 200 \text{ mg}}{\text{have} \rightarrow 1,000 \text{ mg}} \times 3 \text{ mL} \leftarrow \text{quantity}$$

Divide: 200 ÷ 1,000 = 0.2

Multiply: 0.2 × 3 mL = 0.6 mL

No rounding is needed. The patient should be given 0.6 mL.

Dimensional analysis

$$x = \frac{200 \text{ mg}}{1} \times \frac{3 \text{ mL}}{1,000 \text{ mg}}$$

Cancel out duplicate labels, and multiply straight across.

$$x = \frac{200}{1} \times \frac{3 \text{ mL}}{1,000} = \frac{600}{1,000}$$ (multiply the numerators)
(multiply the denominators)

Divide the products: 600 mL ÷ 1,000 = 0.6 mL. No rounding is needed.

5. B

No conversions are necessary for this problem.

Ratio-proportion methods

Means:extremes format:

(number of mg/mL available) 50 mg:1 mL = 75 mg:x mL (ordered mg/unknown mL)

(multiply the means) 75 = 50x (multiply the extremes)

(divide both sides by 50) 75 ÷ 50 = 50x ÷ 50

$$1.5 = x$$

No rounding is needed. The patient should be given 1.5 mL.

Fraction format:

$$\frac{1 \text{ mL}}{50 \text{ mg}} = \frac{x}{75}$$

Cross multiply and solve for *x*.

$$50x = 75$$
$$x = 1.5$$

The patient should be given 1.5 mL.

Formula method

$$\text{desired} \rightarrow \frac{75 \text{ mg}}{50 \text{ mg}} \times 1 \text{ mL} \leftarrow \text{quantity}$$
$$\text{have} \rightarrow$$

Divide: 75 ÷ 50 = 1.5

Multiply: 1.5 × 1 mL = 1.5 mL

Dimensional analysis

$$x = \frac{75 \text{ mg}}{1} \times \frac{1 \text{ mL}}{50 \text{ mg}}$$

Cancel out duplicate labels, and multiply straight across.

$$x = \frac{75}{1} \times \frac{1 \text{ mL}}{50} = \frac{75}{50} \begin{array}{l} \text{(multiply the numerators)} \\ \text{(multiply the denominators)} \end{array}$$

Divide the products: 75 mL ÷ 50 = 1.5 mL.

6. B

No conversions are necessary for this problem.

Ratio-proportion methods

Means : extremes format:

(number of mg/mL available) 50 mg : 1 mL = 100 mg : x mL (ordered mg/unknown mL)
(multiply the means) 100 = 50x (multiply the extremes)
(divide both sides by 50) 100 ÷ 50 = 50x ÷ 50
2 = x

The patient should be given 2 mL.

Fraction format:

$$\frac{1\ mL}{50\ mg} \diagup\!\!\!\!= \frac{x}{100\ mg}$$

Cross multiply and solve for x.

50x = 100
x = 2

The patient should be given 2 mL.

Formula method

$$\frac{desired \rightarrow\ 100\ mg}{have \rightarrow\ 50\ mg} \times 1\ mL \leftarrow quantity$$

Divide: 100 ÷ 50 = 2

Multiply: 2 × 1 mL = 2 mL

Dimensional analysis

$$x = \frac{100\ mg}{1} \times \frac{1\ mL}{50\ mg}$$

Cancel out duplicate labels, and multiply straight across.

$$x = \frac{100}{1} \times \frac{1\ mL}{50} = \frac{100}{50}\ \text{(multiply the numerators)}\ \text{(multiply the denominators)}$$

Divide the products: 100 mL ÷ 50 = 2 mL.

7. A

No conversions are necessary for this problem.

Ratio-proportion methods

Means : extremes format:

(number of mg/mL available) 25 mg : 1 mL = 40 mg : *x* mL (ordered mg/unknown mL)
(multiply the means) 40 = 25*x* (multiply the extremes)
(divide both sides by 25) 40 ÷ 25 = 25*x* ÷ 25
1.6 = *x*

No rounding is needed. The patient should be given 1.6 mL.

Fraction format:

$$\frac{1 \text{ mL}}{25 \text{ mg}} = \frac{x}{40 \text{ mg}}$$

Cross multiply and solve for *x*.

25*x* = 40
x = 1.6

The patient should be given 1.6 mL.

Formula method

$$\frac{\text{desired} \rightarrow 40 \text{ mg}}{\text{have} \rightarrow 25 \text{ mg}} \times 1 \text{ mL} \leftarrow \text{quantity}$$

Divide: 40 ÷ 25 = 1.6

Multiply: 1.6 × 1 mL = 1.6 mL

Dimensional analysis

$$x = \frac{40 \text{ mg}}{1} \times \frac{1 \text{ mL}}{25 \text{ mg}}$$

Cancel out duplicate labels, and multiply straight across.

$$x = \frac{40}{1} \times \frac{1 \text{ mL}}{25} = 75 \text{ (multiply the numerators)} = 25 \text{ (multiply the denominators)}$$

Divide the products: 40 mL ÷ 25 = 1.6 mL.

8. D

No conversions are necessary for this problem.

Ratio-proportion methods

Means : extremes format:

(number of units/mL available) 5,000 units : 1 mL = 800 units : x mL (ordered units/unknown mL)

(multiply the means) 800 = 5,000x (multiply the extremes)

(divide both sides by 5,000) 800 ÷ 5,000 = 5,000x ÷ 5,000

$$0.16 = x$$

No rounding is needed. The patient should be given 0.16 mL.

Fraction format:

$$\frac{1 \text{ mL}}{5,000 \text{ mg}} \diagup\!\!\!\!\diagdown \frac{x}{800 \text{ mg}}$$

Cross multiply and solve for x.

$$5,000x = 800$$
$$x = 0.16$$

The patient should be given 0.16 mL.

Formula method

$$\begin{array}{l} \text{desired} \rightarrow \\ \text{have} \rightarrow \end{array} \frac{800 \text{ units}}{5,000 \text{ units}} \times 1 \text{ mL} \leftarrow \text{quantity}$$

Divide: 800 ÷ 5,000 = 0.16

Multiply: 0.16 × 1 mL = 0.16 mL

Dimensional analysis

$$x = \frac{800 \text{ units}}{1} \times \frac{1 \text{ mL}}{5,000 \text{ units}}$$

Cancel out duplicate labels, and multiply straight across.

$$x = \frac{800}{1} \times \frac{1 \text{ mL}}{5,000} = \begin{array}{l} 800 \quad \text{(multiply the numerators)} \\ 5,000 \quad \text{(multiply the denominators)} \end{array}$$

Divide the products: 800 mL ÷ 5,000 = 0.16 mL.

9. C

Convert 1 g to 1,000 mg (use this conversion for all methods). Disregard the information regarding the volume needed for reconstitution; it is unnecessary information for this type of drug calculation.

Ratio-proportion methods

Means : extremes format:

(number of mg/mL available) 1,000 mg : 2.6 mL = 1,000 mg : x mL (ordered mg/unknown mL)
(multiply the means) 2,600 = 1,000x (multiply the extremes)
(divide both sides by 1,000) 2,600 ÷ 1,000 = 1,000x ÷ 1,000
$$2.6 = x$$

No rounding is needed. The patient should be given 2.6 mL.

Fraction format:

$$\frac{2.6 \text{ mL}}{1,000 \text{ mg}} = \frac{x}{1,000 \text{ mg}}$$

Cross multiply and solve for x.

$$1,000x = 2,600$$
$$x = 2.6$$

The patient should be given 2.6 mL.

Formula method

$$\begin{array}{l}\text{desired} \rightarrow \\ \text{have} \rightarrow \end{array} \frac{1,000 \text{ mg}}{1,000 \text{ mg}} \times 2.6 \text{ mL} \leftarrow \text{quantity}$$

Divide: 1,000 ÷ 1,000 = 1

Multiply: 1 × 2.6 mL = 2.6 mL

Dimensional analysis

$$x = \frac{1,000 \text{ mg}}{1} \times \frac{2.6 \text{ mL}}{1,000 \text{ mg}}$$

Cancel out duplicate labels, and multiply straight across.

$$x = \frac{1,000}{1} \times \frac{2.6 \text{ mL}}{1,000} \begin{array}{l} = 2,600 \quad \text{(multiply the numerators)} \\ = 1,000 \quad \text{(multiply the denominators)} \end{array}$$

Divide the products: 2,600 mL ÷ 1,000 = 2.6 mL.

10. D

Make necessary conversion for this problem: 1 g = 1,000 mg. Disregard the information regarding the volume needed for reconstitution; it is unnecessary information for this type of drug calculation.

Ratio-proportion methods

Means : extremes format:

(number of mg/mL available) 1,000 mg : 2.5 mL = 1,875 mg : x mL (ordered mg/unknown mL)

(multiply the means) 4,687.5 = 1,000x (multiply the extremes)

(divide both sides by 1,000) 4,687.5 ÷ 1,000 = 1,000x ÷ 1,000

$$4.6875 = x$$

Round 4.6875 to the nearest tenth for a final answer of 4.7 mL.

Fraction format:

$$\frac{2.5 \text{ mL}}{1,000 \text{ mg}} = \frac{x}{1,875 \text{ mg}}$$

Cross multiply and solve for x.

$$1,000x = 4,687.5$$
$$x = 4.6875$$

Round 4.6875 to the nearest tenth: 4.7 mL.

Formula method

$$\begin{array}{c} \text{desired} \rightarrow \\ \text{have} \rightarrow \end{array} \frac{1,875 \text{ mg}}{1,000 \text{ mg}} \times 2.5 \text{ mL} \leftarrow \text{quantity}$$

Divide: 1,875 ÷ 1,000 = 1.875

Multiply: 1.875 mL × 2.5 = 4.6875 mL

Round 4.6875 to the nearest tenth: 4.7 mL.

Dimensional analysis

$$x = \frac{1,875 \text{ mg}}{1} \times \frac{2.5 \text{ mL}}{1,000 \text{ mg}}$$

Cancel out duplicate labels, and multiply straight across.

$$x = \frac{1,875}{1} \times \frac{2.5 \text{ mL}}{1,000} = \frac{4,687.5}{1,000} \quad \begin{array}{l} \text{(multiply the numerators)} \\ \text{(multiply the denominators)} \end{array}$$

Divide the products: 4,687.5 ÷ 1,000 = 4.6875.

Round 4.6875 to the nearest tenth: 4.7 mL.

CHAPTER 11

Intravenous Medications

In the hospital setting, most parenteral medications are administered intravenously (IV). Intravenous medications have an extremely short onset, peak, and duration—in some cases, they begin to act in just a few seconds, and their effects can wear off just as quickly. Because of their rapid onset and typically short duration, the rate and frequency used to administer IV medications vary significantly.

Some parenteral medications are administered in doses given over a specific period of time, while others are administered continuously at a set dose or dosage range. Parenteral medications that are administered within a couple of minutes are typically referred to as *IV push medications*. Parenteral medications that are administered over a longer duration of time, such as 20 minutes to 2 hours, may be referred to as *IV piggyback medications* because they are typically infused along with a continuous IV fluid, such as normal saline. In such a case, the continuous IV is referred to as a *maintenance IV* or a carrier. Parenteral medications that are infused continuously and often titrated (adjusted up or down) for a desired effect, such as a target heart rate or blood pressure, are referred to either as *infusions* or *continuous infusions*.

IMPORTANT: Whenever accessing an IV, always clean the port thoroughly according to agency policy, and always flush the site with normal saline to ensure that it is patent before administering fluids or medications through it.

If an IV site is no longer patent, any solution administered through the site may diffuse into surrounding tissue. This diffusion into surrounding tissue is referred to as *infiltration*, and it can be painless or extremely painful. Some medications, particularly IV vasopressors, can cause significant tissue damage and even loss of circulation and tissue necrosis. If an IV site becomes infiltrated, it is important to know which medication(s) have been infused through the site. Be aware of your agency's policy in the event of IV site infiltration.

INTRAVENOUS PUSH (IVP) MEDICATIONS

Intravenous push medications are typically more concentrated than IV piggyback or continuous solutions. While some medications must be administered without being diluted, others require the nurse to dilute them prior to administration. Medications that must be diluted often require a specific diluent—typically normal saline or sterile water. Additionally, some medications may irritate or damage the vessel wall, resulting in phlebitis. These medications are referred to as *vesicants*, and there are often specific policies regarding their administration.

Dosages for IVP medications may be calculated using the ratio-proportion method, formula method, or dimensional analysis. After calculating the dose to be administered, always verify both the rate at which the medication can be administered (e.g., "administer over 2 minutes") and the dilution requirements, if any (e.g., "dilute in 2 mL sterile water").

> **Math Tip:** Because intravenous medications are administered as fluids, the end result of any infusion calculation should be a unit of volume (mL), not weight.

This section reviews how to calculate the IVP rate for every 15 seconds.

Example 1:

> Physician-ordered dose: Diazepam 7.5 mg IVP STAT over 2 minutes
> Dose available: Diazepam 5 mg/mL
> Calculate how much to give every 15 seconds.

First, calculate the total dose to give, using your method of choice. Round answers less than 1 mL to the hundredth and answers greater than 1 mL to the tenth. Regardless of which method you use, the final rounded answer should be 1.5 mL.

Next, determine how much to administer over each minute to reflect the rate ordered, and set up a ratio-proportion equation to determine the push rate.

Means : extremes format

(volume/ordered rate) 1.5 mL : 2 min = x mL : 1 min (unknown volume/1 min)
(multiply the means) $2x = 1.5$ (multiply the extremes)
(divide both sides by 2) $2x \div 2 = 1.5 \div 2$
$x = 0.75$ mL

The nurse should administer the diazepam at a rate of 0.75 mL/minute.

Fraction format

$$\frac{1.5 \text{ mL}}{2 \text{ min}} \bowtie \frac{x}{1 \text{ min}}$$

Cross multiply and solve for x.

$2x = 1.5$

$x = 0.75$ mL

The nurse should administer the diazepam at a rate of 0.75 mL per minute.

Now determine how much to give every 15 seconds.

Means : extremes format

(volume/60 seconds) 0.75 mL : 60 seconds = x mL : 15 seconds (unknown vol/15 seconds)

(multiply the means) $60x = 11.25$ (multiply the extremes)

(divide both sides by 60) $60x \div 60 = 11.25 \div 60$

$x = 0.1875$

Round to 0.19 mL; 0.19 mL should be given every 15 seconds.

Fraction format

$$\frac{0.75 \text{ mL}}{60 \text{ sec}} \bowtie \frac{x}{15 \text{ sec}}$$

Cross multiply and solve for x.

$60x = 11.25$

$x = 0.1875$ mL

Round to 0.19 mL; 0.19 mL should be given every 15 seconds.

Example 2:

Physician-ordered dose: Atenolol 5 mg IVP STAT over 5 minutes
Dose available: Atenolol 5 mg/10 mL
Calculate how much the nurse should give every 15 seconds.

First, calculate how much to give, using your method of choice. Round answers less than 1 mL to the hundredth and answers greater than 1 mL to the tenth. Regardless of the method used, the final rounded answer should be 10 mL.

Next, determine how much to administer over each minute to reflect the rate ordered, and set up a ratio-proportion equation to determine the push rate.

Means : extremes format

(volume/ordered rate in minutes) 10 mL : 5 min = x mL : 1 min (unknown volume/1 min)

(multiply the means) $5x = 10$ (multiply the extremes)

(divide both sides by 5) $5x \div 5 = 10 \div 5$

$x = 2$ mL

The nurse should administer the rate of 2 mL/minute.

Fraction format

$$\frac{10 \text{ mL}}{5 \text{ sec}} \times \frac{x}{1 \text{ min}}$$

Cross multiply and find x.

$5x = 10$

$x = 2$

The nurse should administer at a rate of 2 mL/min.

Determine how much to give every 15 seconds.

Means : extremes format

(volume/60 seconds) 2 mL : 60 sec = x mL : 15 sec (unknown vol/15 seconds)

(multiply the means) $60x = 30$ (multiply the extremes)

(divide both sides by 60) $60x \div 60 = 30 \div 60$

No rounding is necessary; 0.5 mL should be given every 15 seconds.

Fraction format

$$\frac{2 \text{ mL}}{60 \text{ sec}} \times \frac{x}{15 \text{ sec}}$$

Cross multiply and solve for x.

$60x = 30$

$x = 0.5$ mL

0.5 mL should be given every 15 seconds.

Practice 1

Round answers less than 1 mL to the hundredth and answers greater than 1 to the tenth.

1. Physician-ordered dose: Digoxin 0.5 mg IVP STAT over 5 minutes
   Dose available: Digoxin 0.25 mg/mL
   Calculate how much the nurse should give every 15 seconds.

2. Physician-ordered dose: Chlorpromazine hydrochloride 2 mg over 2 minutes
   Dose available: Chlorpromazine hydrochloride 25 mg/mL
   Calculate how much the nurse should give every 15 seconds.

3. Physician-ordered dose: Haloperidol lactate 4 mg IVP over 1.5 minutes
   Dose available: Haloperidol lactate 5 mg/mL
   Calculate how much the nurse should give every 15 seconds.

INTRAVENOUS PIGGYBACK (IVPB) MEDICATIONS

An intravenous piggyback medication is a single dose of medication that is infused over a specified period of time, usually between 20 minutes and 2 hours. When IVPB medications are infused with an electronic pump, infusion rates are usually set in milliliters per hour (mL/hr). Occasionally an IVPB medication may be administered by gravity without the use of an infusion pump. In this case, its infusion rate is calculated in drops per minute.

IMPORTANT: When administering by gravity, it is impossible to deliver an IVPB medication at a precise rate. Gravity administration is also prone to errors—a roller clamp may be bumped, for instance, allowing the medication to flow in much faster than intended. IVPB medication administration by gravity (drops per minute, or gtt/min) is typically reserved for medications with low potential for harm if administered too quickly (some antibiotics) or used in the event of emergency. Always check your agency's policy prior to infusing any medication without an electronic infusion pump.

Calculating IVPB Infusions Using an Electronic Infusion Device

When using an electronic infusion device, a common calculation method is to divide the volume in mL by the infusion time in hours. Most electronic infusion devices can be set to whole numbers only. Because of this, always round answers to the nearest whole number, using the rounding rules discussed in Chapter 3.

> **Math Tip:** To convert minutes to hours, divide the number of minutes by 60.

Example 1:

Physician-ordered dose: Tagamet 300 mg in 100 mL D$_5$W over 30 minutes

Convert minutes to hours: $30 \div 60 = 0.5$. Express the dose as an hourly rate (100 mL/0.5 hr) and convert to a decimal.

$$\frac{\text{(ordered volume in mL)}}{\text{(time in hours)}} \quad \frac{100}{0.5} = 200 \text{ mL/hr}$$

Set the electronic infusion device at 200 mL/hr.

Example 2:

Physician-ordered dose: Erythromycin 250 mg in 100 mL over 45 minutes

Convert minutes to hours: 45 ÷ 60 = 0.75. Express the dose as an hourly rate (100 mL/0.75 hr) and convert to a decimal.

$$\frac{\text{(ordered volume in mL)}}{\text{(time in hours)}} \frac{100}{0.75} = 133.333\ldots$$

Round 133.333… to 133; set the electronic infusion device at 133 mL/hr.

Practice 2

Calculate the following flow rates for practice.

1. Mezlocillin 3 g IVPB in 150 mL NS over 1 hour

2. Geopen 2 g IVPB in 50 mL over 20 minutes

3. KCL 10 mEq in 100 mL $\frac{1}{2}$ NS over 60 minutes

Calculating IVPB Administering by Gravity Infusion

Many medications are infused using IV tubing or administration sets that are manually regulated by the nurse. The standard IV tubing or administration sets that are used for this type of infusion will be either a macrodrop or microdrop tubing. Each IV tubing or administration set delivers a certain number of drops per milliliter. This is called the drop factor. The term *drop factor* is the number of drops the administration set or IV tubing delivers that equals 1 mL. This information is always found on the administration set or IV tubing package. Some manufacturers also include this information on the IV tubing or administration set equipment.

Depending on the manufacturer and the intended use for the tubing, the drop factor on the macrodrop tubing may be 10, 15, or 20 gtts/mL. Macrodrop tubing may also be called macrodrip tubing.

The drop factor on the microdrop tubing is always 60 gtt/mL. Microdrop tubing may also be called minidrip or microdrip tubing.

> **Math Tip:** When using microdrop tubing or administration sets, mL/hr is the same as gtt/min.

First, determine the drop factor for the IV tubing through which the medication will be administered. Multiply the volume in mL by the drop factor, then divide by the ordered infusion time in minutes to get gtt/min.

Example 1:

Kefzol 500 mg in 50 mL over 1 hour. Drop factor = 15.

Convert hours to minutes: 1 hour = 60 minutes.

Multiply the volume in milliliters by the drop factor and divide by the infusion time in minutes.

$$\text{time in minutes} \rightarrow \frac{\overbrace{50 \times 15}^{\text{volume in mL}}}{60} = \leftarrow \text{drop factor}$$

$$\frac{750}{60} = 12.5$$

Round 12.5 to final answer of 13; the medication should infuse at 13 gtt/min.

Example 2:

Gentamicin 150 mg in 200 mL NS over 50 minutes. Drop factor = 20.

No time conversion is necessary.

Multiply the volume in milliliters by the drop factor and divide by the infusion time in minutes.

$$\text{volume in mL} \rightarrow \frac{200 \times 20}{50} = \leftarrow \text{drop factor}$$
$$\text{time in minutes} \rightarrow$$

$$\frac{4,000}{50} = 80$$

The medication should infuse at 80 gtt/min.

Practice 3

Calculate the following flow rates in gtt/min for practice.

1. Zantac 50 mg in 100 mL D_5W over 20 minutes. Drop factor = 15.

2. Timentin 3 g in 75 mL NS over 90 minutes. Drop factor = 60.

3. Chloramphenicol 750 mg in 100 mL lactated Ringer's over 45 minutes. Drop factor = 10.

CONTINUOUS INFUSION MEDICATIONS

Many patients require continuous medication infusions to maintain therapeutic drug blood levels. These medications are absorbed quickly and cannot be recalled. It is vital that these medications be calculated and administered accurately.

This section will discuss administering these drugs via electronic IV pump using the formula method introduced in Chapter 8 ($\frac{D}{H} \times Q = x$). Typically, electronic infusion devices are programmed in mL/hr. Medication orders given in other infusion rates (such as mg/hr, mcg/min, or mL/min) must be converted to mL/hr to be programmed in such devices. Also, because most electronic infusion devices can be set only to whole numbers, all answers must be rounded to the nearest whole number.

Calculating Medications Ordered in Milligrams per Hour

Medications ordered in mg/hr are converted to mL/hr for administration via electronic IV pump, as shown in the following examples.

Example 1:

> Physician-ordered dose: Infuse aminophylline 45 mg/hr
> Dose available: Aminophylline 1 g/1,000 mL 0.45% NS

First, make any necessary conversions between units of measurement. Convert grams to mg so that both doses' weights are in the same unit: 1 g = 1,000 mg.

Then set up the formula.

$$\frac{\text{desired or ordered dose}}{\text{dose available}} \times \text{volume in mL} = \text{mL/hr needed to deliver 45 mg/hr}$$

$$\frac{\text{desired or ordered dose}}{\text{dose available}} \to \frac{45 \text{ mg}}{1,000 \text{ mg}} \times 1,000 \text{ mL} \leftarrow \text{volume dose available}$$

Divide: 45 ÷ 1,000 = 0.045

Multiply: 0.045 × 1,000 = 45 mL/hr

Set the electronic infusion device to 45 mL/hr to administer 45 mg/hr.

Example 2:

Physician-ordered dose: Infuse heparin 1,000 units/hr IV

Dose available: 1,000 mL D₅W with 25,000 units heparin

No conversions are necessary.

$$\frac{\text{desired or ordered dose}}{\text{dose available}} \rightarrow \frac{1,000 \text{ units}}{25,000 \text{ units}} \times 1,000 \text{ mL} \leftarrow \text{volume dose available}$$

Divide: 1,000 ÷ 25,000 = 0.04

Multiply: 0.04 × 1,000 = 40 mL/hr

Set the electronic infusion device to 40 mL/hr to administer 1,000 units/hr.

Practice 4

Calculate the following problems in mL/hr for practice.

1. Physician-ordered dose: Infuse heparin at 1,200 units/hour
   Dose available: Heparin 10,000 units/250 mL D₅W

2. Physician-ordered dose: Infuse aminophylline at 30 mg/hr
   Dose available: Aminophylline 1 g/0.5 L

3. Physician-ordered dose: Infuse regular insulin at 6 units/hr
   Dose available: Regular insulin 250 units/500 mL normal saline

Calculating Medications Ordered in Milligrams per Minute

Medications are sometimes ordered in mL/min. In order to be administered by electronic IV pump, these must also be converted to mL/hr, as shown in the following examples.

Example 1:

Physician-ordered dose: Infuse lidocaine 2 mg/minute
Dose available: Lidocaine 2 g/500 mL

Make any necessary unit conversions: 2 g = 2,000 mg. Then calculate mL/min.

$$\text{desired or ordered dose} \rightarrow \frac{2 \text{ mg}}{2{,}000 \text{ mg}} \times 500 \text{ mL} \leftarrow \text{volume dose available}$$
$$\text{dose available} \rightarrow$$

Divide: 2 ÷ 2,000 = 0.0001

Multiply: 0.0001 × 500 mL = 0.5 mL

So 0.5 mL gives 2 mg, which is the physician-ordered dose per minute. To calculate the dose per hour, multiply by 60: 0.5 mL/min × 60 min/hr = 30 mL/hr.

Set the electronic infusion device at 30 mL/hr to administer 2 mg/minute.

Example 2:

Physician-ordered dose: Infuse pronestyl 3 mg/minute
Dose available: Pronestyl 2 g/250 mL

Make any necessary unit conversions: 2 g = 2,000 mg. Then calculate mL/min.

$$\text{desired or ordered dose} \rightarrow \frac{3 \text{ mg}}{2{,}000 \text{ mg}} \times 250 \text{ mL} \leftarrow \text{volume dose available}$$
$$\text{dose available} \rightarrow$$

Divide: 3 ÷ 2,000 = 0.0015

Multiply: 0.0015 × 250 = 0.375 mL

So 0.375 mL gives 3 mg, which is the physician-ordered dose per minute. To calculate the dose per hour, multiply by 60: 0.375 mL/min × 60 min/hr = 22.5 mL/hr.

Round 22.5 to the nearest whole number: 23 mL/hr.

Set the electronic infusion device at 23 mL/hr to administer 3 mg/minute.

Practice 5

Calculate the following mg/min problems for practice. Express your answers in mL/hr.

1. Physician-ordered dose: Bretylium tosylate 1 mg/min
   Dose available: Bretylium tosylate 2 g/500 mL

2. Physician-ordered dose: Lidocaine 2 mg/min
   Dose available: Lidocaine 2 g/250 mL

3. Physician-ordered dose: Pronestyl 2.5 mg/min
   Dose available: Pronestyl 4 g/500 mL

ANSWERS AND EXPLANATIONS TO PRACTICE EXERCISES

Practice 1

1. 0.1 mL

Using your method of choice, calculate the total volume
to be administered: 2 mL.

Calculate mL/min.

Means : extremes format

(volume/ordered rate in minutes) 2 mL : 5 min = x mL : 1 min (unknown volume/1 min)
(multiply the means) $5x = 2$ (multiply the extremes)
(divide both sides by 5) $5x \div 5 = 2 \div 5$
$x = 0.4$ mL

The nurse should administer at the rate of 0.4 mL/minute.

Fraction format

$$\frac{2 \text{ mL}}{5 \text{ min}} \bowtie \frac{x}{1 \text{ min}}$$

Cross multiply and solve for x.

$5x = 2$
$x = 0.4$ mL

The nurse should administer at a rate of 0.4 mL/minute.

Determine how much to give every 15 seconds.

Means : extremes format

Convert 1 minute to 60 seconds.

(volume/60 seconds) 0.4 mL : 60 sec = x mL : 15 sec (unknown volume/15 seconds)
(multiply the means) $60x = 6$ (multiply the extremes)
(divide both sides by 60) $60x \div 60 = 6 \div 60$
$x = 0.1$ mL

No rounding is necessary; 0.1 mL should be given every
15 seconds.

Fraction format

$$\frac{0.4 \text{ mL}}{60 \text{ sec}} \bowtie \frac{x}{15 \text{ sec}}$$

Cross multiply and solve for x.

$60x = 6$
$x = 0.1$ mL

0.1 mL should be given every 15 seconds.

2. 0.01 mL

Using your method of choice, calculate the total volume to be given: 0.08 mL.

Calculate mL/min.

Means : extremes format

(volume/ordered rate) 0.08 mL : 2 min = x : 1 min (unknown volume/1 min)
(multiply the means) $2x = 0.08$ (multiply the extremes)
(divide both sides by 2) $2x \div 2 = 0.08 \div 2$
$x = 0.04$ mL

The nurse should administer at the rate of 0.04 mL/minute.

Fraction format

$$\frac{0.08 \text{ mL}}{2 \text{ min}} \times \frac{x}{1 \text{ min}}$$

Cross multiply and solve for x.

$2x = 0.08$
$x = 0.04$ mL

The nurse should administer at a rate of 0.04 mL/min.

Determine how much to give every 15 seconds.

Means : extremes format

Convert 1 minute to 60 seconds.

(volume/60 seconds) 0.04 mL : 60 sec = x mL : 15 sec (unknown volume/15 seconds)
(multiply the means) $60x = 0.6$ (multiply the extremes)
(divide both sides by 60) $60x \div 60 = 0.6 \div 60$
$x = 0.01$ mL

No rounding is necessary; 0.01 mL should be given every 15 seconds.

Fraction format

$$\frac{0.04 \text{ mL}}{60 \text{ sec}} \times \frac{x}{15 \text{ sec}}$$

Cross multiply and solve for x.

$60x = 0.6$
$x = 0.01$ mL

The nurse should administer 0.01 mL every 15 seconds.

3. 0.13 mL

Using your method of choice, calculate the total volume to be given: 0.8 mL.

Calculate the mL/min.

Means : extremes format

(volume/ordered rate) 0.8 mL : 1.5 min = x : 1 min (unknown volume/1 min)
(multiply the means) $1.5x = 0.8$ (multiply the extremes)
(divide both sides by 1.5) $1.5x \div 1.5 = 0.8 \div 1.5$
$x = 0.5333... $ mL

Round to 0.53 mL; the nurse should administer at the rate of 0.53 mL/minute.

Fraction format

$$\frac{0.8 \text{ mL}}{1.5 \text{ min}} \diagX \frac{x}{1 \text{ min}}$$

Cross multiply and solve for x.

$1.5x = 0.8$
$x = 0.5333\ldots$ mL

Round to 0.53; the nurse should administer at a rate of 0.53 mL/min.

Determine how much to give every 15 seconds

Means : extremes format

Convert 1 minute to 60 seconds.

(volume/60 seconds) 0.53 mL : 60 sec = x : 15 sec (unknown volume/15 seconds)
(multiply the means) $60x = 7.95$ (multiply the extremes)
(divide both sides by 60) $60x \div 60 = 7.95 \div 60$
$x = 0.1325$ mL

Round to 0.13 mL; the nurse should administer at the rate of 0.13 mL/15 seconds.

Fraction format

$$\frac{0.53 \text{ mL}}{60 \text{ sec}} \diagX \frac{x}{15 \text{ sec}}$$

Cross multiply and solve for x.

$60x = 7.95$
$x = 0.1325$ mL

Round to 0.13; the nurse should administer 0.13 mL every 15 seconds.

Practice 2

1. 150 mL/hr

No time conversion is necessary.

$\dfrac{150}{1}$ ← volume in mL
← time in hours

150 ÷ 1 = 150 mL/hr.

Set the electronic infusion device to 150 mL/hr.

2. 152 mL/hr

Convert minutes to hours: 20 ÷ 60 = 0.333…; round to 0.33 hr. Express the dose as an hourly rate (50 mL/0.33 hr) and convert to a decimal.

$\dfrac{50}{0.33}$ ← volume in mL
← time in hours

50 ÷ 0.33 = 151.5 mL/hr.

Round to 152 mL/hr; set the electronic infusion device to 152 mL/hr.

3. 100 mL/hr

Convert minutes to hours: 60 ÷ 60 = 1 hr.

Express the dose as an hourly rate (100 mL/0.33 hr) and convert to a decimal.

$\dfrac{100}{1}$ ← volume in mL
← time in hours

100 ÷ 1 = 100 mL/hr.

Set the electronic infusion device to 100 mL/hr.

Practice 3

1. 75 gtt/min

volume in mL → $\dfrac{100 \times 15}{20}$ ← drop factor
time in minutes →

$$\dfrac{1,500}{20} = 75$$

The IVPB should infuse at 75 gtt/min.

2. 50 gtt/min

volume in mL → $\dfrac{75 \times 60}{90}$ ← drop factor
time in minutes →

$$\dfrac{4,500}{90} = 50$$

The IVPB should infuse at 50 gtt/min.

3. 22 gtt/min

volume in mL $\rightarrow$ $\dfrac{100 \times 10}{45}$ $\leftarrow$ drop factor
time in minutes $\rightarrow$

$$\frac{1,000}{45} = 22.222\ldots$$

Round to 22 gtt/min; the IVPB should infuse at 22 gtt/min.

Practice 4

1. 30 mL/hr

No conversion between units of measurement is necessary.

desired or ordered dose $\rightarrow$ $\dfrac{1,200 \text{ units}}{10,000 \text{ units}}$ $\times$ 250 mL $\leftarrow$ volume dose available
dose available $\rightarrow$

Divide: $1,200 \div 10,000 = 0.12$

Multiply: $0.12 \times 250 = 30$ mL/hr

Set the electronic infusion device to 30 mL/hr to administer 1,200 units/hr.

2. 15 mL/hr

Convert 1 g to 1,000 mg. Convert 0.5 L to 500 mL.

desired or ordered dose $\rightarrow$ $\dfrac{30 \text{ mg}}{1,000 \text{ mg}}$ $\times$ 500 mL $\leftarrow$ volume dose available
dose available $\rightarrow$

Divide: $30 \div 1,000 = 0.03$

Multiply: $0.03 \times 500 = 15$ mL/hr

Set the electronic infusion device to 15 mL/hr to administer 30 mg/hr.

3. 12 mL/hr

No conversions necessary.

desired or ordered dose $\rightarrow$ $\dfrac{6 \text{ units}}{250 \text{ units}}$ $\times$ 500 mL $\leftarrow$ volume dose available
dose available $\rightarrow$

Divide: $6 \div 250 = 0.024$

Multiply: $0.024 \times 500 = 12$ mL/hr

Set the electronic infusion device to 12 mL/hr to administer 6 units/hr.

Practice 5

1. 15 mL/hr

Convert 2 g to 2,000 mg.

desired or ordered dose → $\dfrac{1 \text{ mg}}{2{,}000 \text{ mg}}$ ← dose available × 500 mL ← volume dose available

Divide: 1 ÷ 2,000 = 0.0005

Multiply: 0.0005 × 500 = 0.25 mL/min

Convert mL/min to mL/hour by multiplying by 60:
0.25 mL/min × 60 min/hr = 15 mL/hr.

Set the electronic infusion device at 15 mL/hr to deliver
1 mg/min.

2. 15 mL/hr

Convert 2 g to 2,000 mg.

desired or ordered dose → $\dfrac{2 \text{ mg}}{2{,}000 \text{ mg}}$ ← dose available × 250 mL ← volume dose available

Divide: 2 ÷ 2,000 = 0.001

Multiply: 0.001 × 250 = 0.25 mL/min

Convert mL/min to mL/hr by multiplying by 60:
0.25 mL/min × 60 min/hr = 15 mL/hr.

Set the electronic infusion device at 15 mL/hr to deliver
2 mg/min.

3. 19 mL/hr

Convert 4 g to 4,000 mg.

desired or ordered dose → $\dfrac{2.5 \text{ mg}}{4{,}000 \text{ mg}}$ ← dose available × 500 mL ← volume dose available

Divide: 2.5 ÷ 4,000 = 0.000625

Multiply: 0.000625 × 500 = 0.3125 mL/min

Convert mL/min to mL/hr by multiplying by 60:
0.3125 mL/min × 60 min/hr = 18.75; round to 19 mL/hr.

Set the electronic infusion device at 19 mL/hr to deliver
2.5 mg/min.

CHAPTER QUIZ

1. Physician-ordered dose: Verapamil hydrochloride 7.5 mg IVP over 3 minutes

   Dose available: Verapamil hydrochloride 2.5 mg/mL

   Calculate how much to give every 15 seconds.

   (A) 0.25 mL   (C) 2.5 mL
   (B) 0.025 mL   (D) .025 mL

2. Physician-ordered dose: Warfarin sodium 3 mg IVP daily over 1 minute

   Dose available: Warfarin sodium 2 mg/mL

   Calculate how much to give every 15 seconds.

   (A) 1.5 mL   (C) 0.15 mL
   (B) 0.38 mL   (D) 0.04 mL

3. Physician-ordered dose: Infuse meropenem 1 g/100 mL D_5W over 20 minutes

   What flow rate should the electronic infusion device be set at?

   (A) 300 mL/hr   (C) 303 mL/hr
   (B) 100 mL/hr   (D) 30 mL/hr

4. Physician-ordered dose: Infuse methicillin
   1.5 g in 75 mL NS over 30 minutes

   What flow rate should the electronic infusion
   device be set at?

   (A) 150 mL/hr   (C) 15 mL/hr

   (B) 75 mL/hr   (D) 200 mL/hr

5. Physician-ordered dose: Infuse jenamicin
   180 mg/50 mL D_5W over 30 minutes

   Drop factor = 15

   What is the flow rate?

   (A) 25 mL/hr   (C) 3 gtt/min

   (B) 3 mL/hr   (D) 25 gtt/min

6. Physician-ordered dose: Infuse penicillin G
   2,000,000 units/50 mL D_5W over 45 minutes

   Drop factor = 60

   What is the flow rate?

   (A) 50 mL/hr   (C) 66 gtt/min

   (B) 66 mL/hr   (D) 67 gtt/min

7. Physician-ordered dose: Infuse heparin at 700 units/hr IV infusion

   Dose available: Heparin 20,000 units/500 mL

   What is the flow rate?

   (A) 18 mL/hr   (C) 18 gtt/min
   (B) 17.5 mL/hr   (D) 17 gtt/min

8. Physician-ordered dose: Infuse aminophylline at 60 mg/hr

   Dose available: Aminophylline 500 mg/250 mL $\frac{1}{2}$ NS

   What is the flow rate?

   (A) 60 mL/hr   (C) 30 mL/hr
   (B) 60 gtt/min   (D) 30 gtt/min

9. Physician-ordered dose: Infuse pronestyl 2 mg/min

   Dose available: Pronestyl 1 g/250 mL

   What is the flow rate?

   (A) 15 mL/hr   (C) 0.5 mL/hr
   (B) 50 mL/hr   (D) 30 mL/hr

10. Physician-ordered dose: Lidocaine 4 mg/min

   Dose available: Lidocaine 2 g/500 mL

   What is the flow rate?

   (A) 30 mL/hr   (C) 20 mL/hr
   (B) 60 mL/hr   (D) 40 mL/hr

ANSWERS AND EXPLANATIONS

1.   A

Use method of choice to solve for volume to administer:
3 mL.

Means : extremes format

Calculate mL/min.

(volume ordered rate in minutes) 3 mL:3 min = x mL:1 min (unknown volume/1 min)
(multiply the means) $3x = 3$ (multiply the extremes)
(divide both sides by 3) $3x \div 3 = 3 \div 3$
$x = 1$ mL/minute

Determine how much to give every 15 seconds.

Convert 1 minute to 60 seconds.

(volume/60 seconds) 1 mL:60 sec = x mL:15 sec (unknown volume/15 seconds)
$60x = 15$
$60x \div 60 = 15 \div 60$
$x = 0.25$

No rounding is necessary; 0.25 mL should be administered
every 15 seconds.

Fraction format

Calculate mL/min.

$$\frac{3 \text{ mL}}{3 \text{ min}} \times \frac{x \text{ mL}}{1 \text{ min}}$$

Cross multiply and solve for x.

$3x = 3$
$x = 1$ mL/min

Determine how much to give every 15 seconds.

Convert 1 minute to 60 seconds.

$$\frac{1 \text{ mL}}{60 \text{ sec}} \times \frac{x}{15 \text{ sec}}$$

Cross multiply and solve for x.

$60x = 15$
$x = 0.25$ mL

0.25 mL should be administered every 15 seconds.

2. B

Use method of choice to solve for volume to administer:
1.5 mL.

Means : extremes format

Calculate mL/min.

> (rate in minutes) 1.5 mL : 1 min = x mL : 1 min (unknown volume/1 min)
> (multiply the means) $1x = 1.5$ (multiply the extremes)
> (divide both sides by 1) $1x \div 1 = 1.5 \div 1$
> $x = 1.5$ mL

1.5 mL should be administered every minute.

Determine how much to give every 15 seconds.

Convert 1 minute to 60 seconds.

> (volume/60 seconds) 1.5 mL : 60 sec = x mL : 15 sec (unknown volume/15 seconds)
> $60x = 22.5$
> $60x \div 60 = 22.5 \div 60$
> $x = 0.375$ mL

Round to 0.38; 0.38 mL should be administered every
15 seconds.

Fraction format

Calculate mL/min.

> $\dfrac{1.5 \text{ mL}}{1 \text{ min}} \underset{\times}{=} \dfrac{x \text{ mL}}{1 \text{ min}}$

Cross multiply and solve for x.

> $1x = 1.5$
> $x = 1.5$ mL

1.5 mL should be administered every minute.

Determine how much to give every 15 seconds.

Convert 1 minute to 60 seconds.

> $\dfrac{1.5 \text{ mL}}{60 \text{ sec}} \underset{\times}{=} \dfrac{x}{15 \text{ sec}}$

Cross multiply and solve for x.

> $60x = 22.5$
> $x = 0.375$ mL

Round to 0.38; 0.38 mL should be administered every
15 seconds.

3. C

Convert 20 minutes to hours: 20 ÷ 60 = 0.333...; round to 0.33.

Express the dose as an hourly rate (100 mL/0.33 hr) and convert to a decimal.

$\dfrac{100}{0.33}$ ← volume in mL
← time in hours

100 ÷ 0.33 = 303.0303... mL/hr

Round to 303 mL; set the electronic infusion device to 303 mL/hr.

4. A

Convert 30 minutes to hours: 30 ÷ 60 = 0.5.

Express the dose as an hourly rate (75 mL/0.5 hr) and convert to a decimal.

$\dfrac{75}{0.5}$ ← volume in mL
← time in hours

75 ÷ 0.5 = 150 mL/hr

Set the electronic infusion device to 150 mL/hr.

5. D

Multiply the volume in milliliters by the drop factor and divide by the infusion time in minutes.

volume in mL → $\dfrac{50 \times 15}{30}$ ← drop factor
time in minutes →

$\dfrac{750}{30} = 25$

The medication should infuse at 25 gtt/min.

6. D

Multiply the volume in milliliters by the drop factor and divide by the infusion time in minutes.

volume in mL → $\dfrac{50 \times 60}{45}$ ← drop factor
time in minutes →

$\dfrac{3,000}{45} = 66.666...$

Round to 67 gtt/min; the medication should infuse at 67 gtt/min.

7. A

No conversions needed. Calculate mL/min.

desired or ordered dose → $\dfrac{700 \text{ units}}{20{,}000 \text{ units}}$ × 500 mL ← volume dose available
(dose available →)

Divide: 700 ÷ 20,000 = 0.035

Multiply: 0.035 × 500 = 17.5 mL/hr

Round to 18 mL/hr; set the electronic infusion device at
18 mL/hr to administer 700 units/hr.

8. C

No conversions needed. Calculate mL/min.

desired or ordered dose → $\dfrac{60 \text{ mg}}{500 \text{ mg}}$ × 250 mL ← volume dose available
(dose available →)

Divide: 60 ÷ 500 = 0.24

Multiply: 0.24 × 25 = 30 mL/hr

Set the electronic infusion device at 30 mL/hr to administer
60 mg/hr.

9. D

Make any necessary conversions: 1 g = 1,000 mg. Calculate mL/min.

desired or ordered dose → $\dfrac{2 \text{ mg}}{1{,}000 \text{ mg}}$ × 250 mL ← volume dose available
(dose available →)

Divide: 2 ÷ 1,000 = 0.002

Multiply: 0.002 × 250 = 0.5 mL/min

Convert mL/min to mL/hr by multiplying by 60:
0.5 mL/min × 60 min/hr = 30 mL/hr.

Set the electronic infusion device at 30 mL/hr to administer
2 mg/min.

10. B

Make any necessary conversions: 2 g = 2,000 mg. Calculate mL/min.

desired or ordered dose → $\dfrac{4 \text{ mg}}{2{,}000 \text{ mg}}$ × 500 mL ← volume dose available
(dose available →)

Divide: 4 ÷ 2,000 = 0.002

Multiply: 0.002 × 500 = 1 mL/min

Convert mL/min to mL/hr by multiplying by 60:
1 mL/min × 60 min/hr = 60 mL/hr.

Set the electronic infusion device at 60 mL/hr to administer
4 mg/min.

CHAPTER 12

Age-Specific Considerations

Children, adults, and older adults metabolize drugs differently. Furthermore, in terms of body composition these three populations tend to have different percentages of adipose and total body water. While many parenteral drugs are distributed and metabolized in much the same way as oral medications, some require more patient-specific dosing. Many vasoactive medications, chemotherapy drugs, and sedatives have a predefined infusion range intended to achieve a specific concentration within the body. Dopamine, for instance, causes an increase in heart rate and blood pressure, and its effects amplify at higher concentrations. In cases where a drug must penetrate certain tissues in the body to achieve its therapeutic effect, a larger body requires a higher total dose of medication. Because of these differences, many medications are dosed based on either body weight or body surface area.

> **Math Tip:** For accurate dosage calculation rounding, do not use a calculator with an automatic rounding feature; or program the calculator to turn off that feature.

CALCULATING MEDICATIONS BASED ON WEIGHT

Many medications are calculated and administered based on the patient's weight in kilograms. The first step to solving these problems is to obtain an accurate patient weight. If necessary, convert weights obtained in pounds to kilograms. To convert pounds to kilograms, divide the number of pounds by 2.2. The next step is to multiply the ordered dose per kilogram by the number of kilograms of patient weight. This will be the total ordered dose. The problem may now be solved using ratio-proportion, the formula method, or dimensional analysis.

> **Math Tip:**
> 2.2 lb = 1 kg
> 1 inch = 2.5 cm

Example 1:

The patient is a 60-year-old man. His weight is 158 lb.
Physician-ordered dose: Tobramycin sulfate 3 mg/kg IM tid
Dose available: Tobramycin sulfate 80 mg/2 mL

Convert 158 lb to kg: $158 \div 2.2 = 71.8181$. Round weights to the nearest tenth to get 71.8 kg. Since the order is 3 mg per 1 kg, the nurse must multiply the weight of 71.8 by 3 mg to get the total ordered dose: $71.8 \times 3 = 215.4$ mg. Using your method of choice, calculate how much the nurse should administer.

Means : extremes format

The dosages in this problem use the same units of measurement, so no conversions are necessary.

(mg/mL available) 80 mg : 2 mL = 215.4 mg : x mL (ordered dose/unknown mL)
(multiply the means) $430.8 = 80x$ (multiply the extremes)
(divide both sides by 80) $430.8 \div 80 = 80x \div 80$
$$5.385 = x$$

Round to the tenth to get 5.4 mL.

The nurse should administer 5.4 mL to the patient.

Fraction format

No conversions are necessary.

$$\frac{2 \text{ mL}}{80 \text{ mg}} \diagtimes \frac{x}{215.4 \text{ mg}}$$

Cross multiply and solve for x.

$80x = 430.8$
$x = 5.385$ mL

Round to the nearest tenth to get 5.4 mL. The nurse should administer 5.4 mL to the patient.

Formula method

No conversions are necessary.

$$\text{desired} \rightarrow \frac{215.4 \text{ mg}}{80 \text{ mg}} \times 2 \text{ mL} \leftarrow \text{quantity}$$
$$\text{have} \rightarrow$$

Divide: $215.4 \div 80 = 5.385$

Multiply: $5.385 \times 2 \text{ mL} = 10.770 \text{ mL}$

Dimensional analysis

No conversions are necessary. Set up the problem, ensuring that any duplicate units appear in both the numerator and denominator.

$$x = \frac{\overset{\text{(ordered dose)}}{\text{Desired}}}{1 \text{ (constant)}} \times \frac{\overset{\text{(available dose)}}{\text{Equivalent (unit different from Desired)}}}{\text{Equivalent (unit same as Desired)}}$$

$$x = \frac{215.4 \text{ mg}}{1} \times \frac{2 \text{ mL}}{80 \text{ mg}}$$

Cancel out the units that appear in both the numerator and denominator, and multiply straight across.

$$x = \frac{2 \text{ mL}}{80} \times \frac{215.4}{1} = \begin{matrix} 430.8 & \text{(multiply the numerators)} \\ 80 & \text{(multiply the denominators)} \end{matrix}$$

Divide the products: $430.8 \text{ mL} \div 80 = 5.385 \text{ mL}$.

Round to the nearest tenth: $x = 5.4 \text{ mL}$.

The nurse should administer 5.4 mL to the patient.

Example 2:

> The patient is 12 months old. Her weight is 22 lb.
> Physician-ordered dose: Oxacillin sodium 50 mg/kg po every 6 hours
> Dose available: Oxacillin sodium 250 mg/5 mL

Convert 22 lb to kg: $22 \div 2.2 = 10$. No rounding is necessary. Since the order is 50 mg per 1 kg, the nurse must multiply the weight of 10 kg by 50 mg to get the total ordered dose: $10 \times 50 = 500$ mg. Using your method of choice, calculate how much the nurse should administer for each dose. The ordered dose and the dose available in this problem use the same units of measurement (mg), so no conversions are necessary.

Means : extremes format

(mg/mL available) 250 mg : 5 mL = 500 mg : x mL (ordered dose/unknown mL)
(multiply the means) 2,500 = 250x (multiply the extremes)
(divide both sides by 80) 2,500 ÷ 250 = 250x ÷ 250

$$10 = x$$

The nurse should administer 10 mL to the patient.

Fraction format

$$\frac{5 \text{ mL}}{250 \text{ sec}} \diagup\!\!\!\!\diagdown \frac{x}{500 \text{ mg}}$$

Cross multiply and solve for x.

$$250x = 2,500$$
$$x = 10 \text{ mL}$$

The nurse should administer 10 mL to the patient.

Formula method

$$\begin{array}{c} \text{desired} \rightarrow \\ \text{have} \rightarrow \end{array} \frac{500 \text{ mg}}{250 \text{ mg}} \times 5 \text{ mL} \leftarrow \text{quantity}$$

Divide: 500 ÷ 250 = 2

Multiply: 2 × 5 mL = 10 mL

The nurse should administer 10 mL to the patient.

Dimensional analysis

$$x = \frac{500 \text{ mg}}{1} \times \frac{5 \text{ mL}}{250 \text{ mg}}$$

Cancel out duplicate labels, and multiply straight across.

$$x = \frac{500}{1} \times \frac{5 \text{ mL}}{250} = \frac{2,500}{250} \quad \begin{array}{l} \text{(multiply the numerators)} \\ \text{(multiply the denominators)} \end{array}$$

Divide the products: 2,500 ÷ 250 = 10.

The nurse should administer 10 mL to the patient.

Practice 1

Using your method of choice, solve the following problems. Round weights to the nearest tenth. Round answers less than 1 mL to the hundredth and answers greater than 1 mL to the nearest tenth.

1. The patient is 74 years old and has renal disease. His weight is 165 lb.
   Physician-ordered dose: Amikacin sulfate 7.5 mg/kg IM bid
   Dose available: Amikacin sulfate 250 mg/mL
   How much should the nurse administer?

2. The patient is 9 years old and has asthma. Her weight is 55 lb.
   Physician-ordered dose: Aminophylline 3 mg/kg po tid
   Dose available: Aminophylline 105 mg/5 mL
   How much should the nurse administer?

CALCULATING CONTINUOUS INFUSION RATES BASED ON WEIGHT

Vasoactive and sedating medications exert a mild effect at low doses and a profound effect at high doses. These medications are often titrated until the desired effect is achieved. Epinephrine, for instance, is typically titrated to maintain a target systolic blood pressure or mean arterial pressure. Propofol is a general anesthetic that can be titrated for moderate or heavy sedation. To be administered safely, these continuous infusions are infused at rates that are specific to the patient's weight. Weight-specific infused medications should always be administered with an electronic infusion pump to ensure precise monitoring and control at all times. Electronic infusion pumps are programmed in mL/hr using whole numbers. Many modern pumps now have drug libraries and may be programmed in mcg/kg/min, but the nurse must always confirm these values by manual calculation.

First, convert the available dose from mg/mL to mcg/mL by multiplying by 1,000 as shown.

$$\frac{\text{mg in solution} \times 1{,}000}{\text{total volume in mL}}$$

Second, calculate the mL/hr to set the electronic infusion device using the following formula.

$$\frac{(\text{ordered mcg/kg/min}) \times (60 \text{ min/hr}) \times (\text{wt in kg})}{(\text{available mcg/mL})}$$

Example 1:

Physician-ordered dose: Infuse dopamine hydrochloride 5 mcg/kg/min
Dose available: Dopamine hydrochloride 400 mg/250 mL D_5W
Patient weight: 175 lb

Convert the patient's weight from pounds to kilograms and round to the tenth:

$175 \div 2.2 = 79.5$ kg

Convert the available dose from mg/mL to mcg/mL by multiplying by 1,000.

$$\frac{\text{mg in solution} \times 1{,}000}{\text{total volume in mL}} \rightarrow \frac{400 \times 1{,}000}{250} = \frac{400{,}000 \text{ mcg}}{250 \text{ mL}}$$

Reduce this fraction to lowest terms: 400,000 mcg ÷ 250 mL = 1,600 mcg/mL. There are 1,600 mcg per mL.

Set up the formula to determine mL/hr to equal mcg/kg/min.

$$\frac{(\text{ordered mcg/kg/min}) \times (60 \text{ min/hr}) \times (\text{wt in kg})}{(\text{available mcg/mL})}$$

Now fill in the values and cross off the labels.

$$\frac{5\ mcg/kg/min \times 60\ min/hr \times 79.5\ kg}{1,600\ mcg/mL}$$

$$\frac{5 \times 60 \times 79.5}{1,600} = \frac{23,850}{1,600} = 14.9$$

Round to the nearest whole number. The nurse should set the electronic infusion device at 15 mL/hr to deliver 5 mcg/kg/min.

Example 2:

Physician-ordered dose: Infuse nipride 2 mcg/kg/min

Dose available: Nipride 50 mg/250 mL D₅W

Patient weight: 140 lb

Convert the patient's weight from pounds to kilograms and round to the tenth:

$$140 \div 2.2 = 63.6\ kg$$

Convert the available dose from mg/mL to mcg/mL by multiplying by 1,000.

$$\frac{mg\ in\ solution}{total\ volume\ in\ mL} \times 1,000 \rightarrow \frac{50 \times 1,000}{250} = \frac{50,000\ mcg}{250\ mL}$$

Reduce to lowest terms: 50,000 mcg ÷ 250 mL = 200 mcg/mL. There are 200 mcg per mL.

Set up the formula to determine mL/hr to equal mcg/kg/min. Then cross off the labels, multiply, and reduce to lowest terms.

$$\frac{2\ mcg/kg/min \times 60\ min/hr \times 63.6\ kg}{200\ mcg/mL}$$

$$\frac{2 \times 60 \times 63.6}{200} = \frac{7,632}{200} = 38.16$$

Round to the nearest whole number. The nurse should set the electronic infusion device at 38 mL/hr to deliver 2 mcg/kg/min.

Practice 2

Solve the following problems for practice. Round weights to the tenth and infusion rates to the nearest whole number.

1. Physician-ordered dose: Infuse dobutamine hydrochloride at 3 mcg/kg/min.
    Dose available: Dobutamine hydrochloride 250 mg/500 mL
    Patient weight: 132 lb
    At what mL/hr rate should the nurse set the electronic infusion device?

2. Physician-ordered dose: Infuse dopamine hydrochloride at 2.5 mcg/kg/min.
    Dose available: Dopamine hydrochloride 200 mg/250 mL D₅W
    Patient weight: 180 lb
    At what mL/hr rate should the nurse set the electronic infusion device?

MEDICATION DOSES BASED ON BODY SURFACE AREA (BSA)

Body surface area is calculated in square meters, or m². Calculating medications based on BSA is frequently used for pediatric and fragile adult patients and those taking certain medications. Frequently, these types of patients are at high risk and require a more precise method of medication calculation. The most accurate weight to use for BSA calculations is the lean body weight—the body weight prior to any edema. It is best to measure the patient for the correct height, as many children may have grown since last measured, and many elderly may have lost height due to osteoporosis.

Several formulas may be used for calculating BSA. This section will focus on calculating BSA and how to determine the ordered dose using the *Mosteller formula* in the metric format. This formula is easy to remember and can be calculated with a basic function calculator. This formula is the same for adults and pediatric patients.

Because this formula uses the metric system, the nurse will have to convert weights to kilograms and heights to centimeters. Calculating BSA with this formula involves square roots. The nurse should always use a reliable calculator for these calculations, and it is always a good habit to double-check all calculations for accuracy.

Nurses performing this type of calculation should be aware of facility policy and use that facility's approved calculation. Some facilities use a nomogram to perform these calculations. If so, then it is essential that the nurse use the appropriate nomogram for each individual patient.

When correctly executed, both methods are accurate. After the ordered dose is determined, the amount to be administered may be calculated by using ratio-proportion, formula, or dimensional analysis method.

> **Math Tip:** To ensure an accurate medication dosage calculation, only use the pediatric nomogram for children and the adult nomogram for adults.

CALCULATING MEDICATION DOSES BASED ON BODY SURFACE AREA

Example 1:

Physician-ordered dose: Allopurinol 400 mg/m²/day IV daily
Dose available: Allopurinol 500 mg/30 mL
Patient weight: 166 lb
Patient height: 65 inches

Calculate the ordered dose.

After converting the patient's weight and height to metric, use the following formula to calculate BSA.

$$BSA = \sqrt{\frac{\text{height in cm} \times \text{weight in kg}}{3{,}600 \text{ (constant) m}^2 \text{ (square meters)}}}$$

> **Math Tip:** To enter the calculation into a calculator, follow these steps: (1) multiply height in cm by weight in kg; (2) divide by 3,600; and (3) press the square root symbol on the calculator. Then round to the hundredth. The result is the patient's body surface area in square meters.

STEP 1: Convert patient weight to kg and round to the tenth:
$166 \div 2.2 = 75.4545 \rightarrow 75.5$ kg.

STEP 2: Convert patient height to cm and round to the tenth:
$65 \times 2.5 = 162.5$ cm (no rounding needed).

STEP 3: Calculate patient BSA.

$$BSA = \sqrt{\frac{162.5 \text{ cm} \times 7.5 \text{ kg}}{3{,}600 \text{ (constant) m}^2 \text{ (square meters)}}}$$

The result is 1.846073. Round to the hundredth: 1.85. The patient's BSA is 1.85 m².

STEP 4: Calculate the desired dose.

Multiply the BSA by the ordered dose: $1.85 \times 400 = 740$ mg. The total ordered dose is 740 mg. The nurse should use a reliable source to confirm that the dose is within the medication's recommended range.

Example 2:

Physician-ordered dose: sargramostim 250 mcg/m²/day
Patient weight: 175 lb
Patient height: 73 inches

Calculate the ordered dose.

STEP 1: Convert patient weight to kg and round to the tenth:
$175 \div 2.2 = 79.5454 \rightarrow 79.5$ kg.

STEP 2: Convert patient height to cm and round to the tenth:
$73 \times 2.5 = 182.5$ cm (no rounding needed).

STEP 3: Calculate patient BSA.

$$BSA = \sqrt{\frac{182.5 \text{ cm} \times 79.5 \text{ kg}}{3{,}600 \text{ m}^2}}$$

The result is 2.0075378. Round to the hundredth: 2.01. The patient's BSA is 2.01 m².

STEP 4: Calculate the desired dose.

Multiply the BSA by the ordered dose: $2.01 \times 250 = 502.5$ mcg. The total ordered dose is 502.5 mcg (no rounding needed). The nurse should use a reliable source to confirm that the dose is within the recommended range.

Example 3:

Physician-ordered dose: Pentamidine 100 mg/m²/daily for 5 days
Patient weight: 35 lb
Patient height: 36 inches

Calculate the daily dose.

STEP 1: Convert patient weight to kg and round to the tenth: $35 \div 2.2 = 15.9$ kg.

STEP 2: Convert patient height to cm and round to the tenth: $36 \times 2.5 = 90$ cm.

STEP 3: Calculate patient BSA.

$$BSA = \sqrt{\frac{90 \text{ cm} \times 15.9 \text{ kg}}{3{,}600 \text{ m}^2}}$$

The result is 0.6304. Round to the hundredth: 0.63. The patient's BSA is 0.63 m².

STEP 4: Calculate the desired dose.

Multiply the BSA by the ordered dose: $0.63 \times 100 = 63$ mg. The total ordered dose is 63 mg. The nurse should use a reliable source to confirm that the dose is within the recommend range.

Practice 3

Solve the following problems based on BSA. Round weights and heights to the tenth. Round BSA to the hundredth. Round doses greater than 1 mL to the tenth and doses less than 1 mL to the hundredth.

1. Physician-ordered dose: Etoposide 35 mg/m²/day today
   Patient weight: 100 lb
   Patient height: 56 inches
   Calculate the ordered dose.

2. Physician-ordered dose: Mitomycin 20 mg/m² today
   Patient weight: 200 lb
   Patient height: 63 inches
   Calculate the ordered dose.

ANSWERS AND EXPLANATIONS TO PRACTICE EXERCISES

Practice 1

1. 2.3 mL

Convert 165 lb to kg: 165 ÷ 2.2 = 75 kg.

Multiply 75 kg by 7.5 mg per kg to get a total ordered dose of 562.5 mg.

The patient's weight in kg is already stated to the tenth, so no rounding is needed. The ordered dose and the dose available in this problem use the same unit of measurement (mg), so no conversions are necessary.

Means : extremes format

(mg/mL available) 250 mg : 1 mL = 562.5 mg : x mL (ordered dose/unknown mL)
(multiply the means) 562.5 = 250x (multiply the extremes)
(divide both sides by 250) 562.5 ÷ 250 = 250x ÷ 250
$$2.25 = x$$

Round to 2.3. The nurse should administer 2.3 mL to the patient.

Fraction format

$$\frac{1 \text{ mL}}{250 \text{ mg}} \times \frac{x}{562.5 \text{ mg}}$$

Cross multiply and find x.

$$250x = 562.5$$
$$x = 2.25 \text{ mL}$$

Round to 2.3. The nurse should administer 2.3 mL to the patient.

Formula method

$$\text{desired} \rightarrow \frac{562.5 \text{ mg}}{250 \text{ mg}} \times 1 \text{ mL} \leftarrow \text{quantity}$$
$$\text{have} \rightarrow$$

Divide: 562.5 ÷ 250 = 2.25

Multiply: 2.25 × 1 mL = 2.25 mL

Round to 2.3. The nurse should administer 2.3 mL to the patient.

Dimensional analysis

$$x = \frac{562.5 \text{ mg}}{1} \times \frac{1 \text{ mL}}{250 \text{ mg}}$$

Cancel out the units that appear in both the numerator and denominator, and multiply straight across.

$$x = \frac{562.5}{1} \times \frac{1 \text{ mL}}{250} = \frac{562.5}{250} \quad \text{(multiply the numerators)} \quad \text{(multiply the denominators)}$$

Divide the products: $562.5 \div 250 = 2.25$.

Round to the nearest tenth: $x = 2.3$ mL.

The nurse should administer 2.3 mL to the patient.

2.   3.6 mL

Convert 55 lb to kg: $55 \div 2.2 = 25$ kg.

Multiply 25 kg by 3 mg per kg to get a total ordered dose of 75 mg.

No rounding is needed to the patient's weight in kg. The ordered dose and the dose available use the same unit of measurement (mg), so no conversions are necessary.

Means : extremes format

(number of mg/mL available) 105 mg : 5 mL = 75 mg : x mL (ordered mg/unknown mL)
(multiply the means) $375 = 105x$ (multiply the extremes)
(divide both sides by 105) $375 \div 105 = 105x \div 105$
$3.57142857... = x$

Round $3.57142857...$ to the nearest tenth: $x = 3.6$ mL.
The nurse should administer 3.6 mL to the patient.

Fraction format

$$\frac{5 \text{ mL}}{105 \text{ mg}} \times \frac{1 \text{ mL}}{75 \text{ mg}}$$

Cross multiply and find x.

$$105x = 375$$
$$x = 3.57142857... \text{ mL}$$

Round to the nearest tenth: 3.6 mL.

The nurse should administer 3.6 mL to the patient.

Formula method

$$\text{desired} \rightarrow \frac{75 \text{ mg}}{105 \text{ mg}} \times 1 \text{ mL} \leftarrow \text{quantity}$$
$$\text{have} \rightarrow$$

Divide: $75 \div 105 = 3.57142857\ldots$

Multiply: $3.57142857\ldots \times 1 \text{ mL} = 3.57142857\ldots \text{ mL}$.

Round to 3.6. The nurse should administer 3.6 mL.

Dimensional analysis

$$x = \frac{75 \text{ mg}}{1} \times \frac{5 \text{ mL}}{105 \text{ mg}}$$

Cancel out the duplicate labels, and multiply straight across.

$$x = \frac{75}{1} \times \frac{5 \text{ mL}}{105} = \frac{375 \text{ mL}}{105} \quad \begin{array}{l}\text{(multiply the numerators)}\\ \text{(multiply the denominators)}\end{array}$$

Divide the products: $375 \div 105 = 3.57142857\ldots \text{ mL}$.

Round to 3.6 mL.

Practice 2

1. 22 mL/hr

Convert the patient's weight from pounds to kilograms:
$132 \div 2.2 = 60$ kg. No rounding is needed.

Convert the available dose from mg/mL to mcg/mL
(multiply by 1,000) and reduce to lowest terms.

$$\frac{\text{mg in solution} \times 1{,}000}{\text{total volume in mL}} \rightarrow \frac{250 \times 1{,}000}{500} = \frac{250{,}000 \text{ mcg}}{500 \text{ mL}} = \frac{500 \text{ mcg}}{1 \text{ mL}}$$

There are 500 mcg per mL.

Set up the formula to determine mL/hr to equal mcg/kg/min.

$$\frac{(\text{ordered mcg/kg/min}) \times (60 \text{ min/hr}) \times (\text{wt in kg})}{(\text{available mcg/mL})}$$

$$\frac{3 \text{ mcg/kg/min} \times 60 \text{ min/hr} \times 60 \text{ kg}}{500 \text{ mcg/mL}}$$

Cross off the labels, multiply, and reduce to lowest terms.

$$\frac{3 \times 60 \times 60}{500} = \frac{10{,}800}{500} = 21.6$$

Round 21.6 to the nearest whole number: 22. The nurse
should set the electronic infusion device at 22 mL/hr to
deliver 3 mcg/kg/min.

2. 15 mL/hr

Convert the patient's weight from pounds to kilograms and round to the tenth: $180 \div 2.2 = 81.8$ kg.

Convert the available dose from mg/mL to mcg/mL (multiply by 1,000) and reduce to lowest terms.

$$\frac{\text{mg in solution} \times 1,000 \rightarrow}{\text{total volume in mL} \rightarrow} \frac{200 \times 1,000}{250} = \frac{200,000 \text{ mcg}}{250 \text{ mL}} = \frac{800 \text{ mcg}}{\text{mL}}$$

There are 800 mcg per mL.

Set up the equation to determine mL/hr to equal mcg/kg/min.

$$\frac{2.5 \text{ mcg/kg/min} \times 60 \text{ min/hr} \times 81.8 \text{ kg}}{800 \text{ mcg/mL}}$$

Cross off the labels, multiply, and reduce to lowest terms.

$$\frac{2.5 \times 60 \times 81.8}{800} = \frac{12,270}{800} = 15.3375$$

Round to the nearest whole number. The nurse should set the electronic infusion device at 15 mL/hr to deliver 2.5 mcg/kg/min.

Practice 3

1. 46.6 mg

STEP 1: Convert patient weight to kg and round to the tenth: $100 \div 2.2 = 45.4545 \rightarrow 45.5$ kg.

STEP 2: Convert patient height to cm and round to the tenth: $56 \times 2.5 = 140$ cm (no rounding needed).

STEP 3: Calculate patient BSA.

$$\text{BSA} = \sqrt{\frac{140 \text{ cm} \times 45.5 \text{ kg}}{3,600 \text{ m}^2}}$$

The patient's BSA is 1.330204. Round to the hundredth: 1.33 m^2.

STEP 4: Calculate the desired dose.

Multiply the BSA by the ordered dose: $1.33 \times 35 = 46.55$.

Round to the tenth: 46.6. The total ordered dose is 46.6 mg/day. The nurse should use a reliable source to confirm that the dose is within the recommend range and then administer as ordered.

2. 39.8 mg

STEP 1: Convert patient weight to kg and round to the tenth: $200 \div 2.2 = 90.90 \rightarrow 90.9$ kg.

STEP 2: Convert patient height to cm and round to the tenth: $63 \times 2.5 = 157.5$ cm (no rounding needed).

STEP 3: Calculate patient BSA.

$$BSA = \sqrt{\frac{157.5 \text{ cm} \times 90.9 \text{ kg}}{3{,}600 \text{ m}^2}}$$

The patient's BSA is 1.994. Round to 1.99 m².

STEP 4: Calculate the desired dose.

Multiply the BSA by the ordered dose: $1.99 \times 20 = 39.8$ (no rounding needed). The total ordered dose is 39.8 mg/day. The nurse should use a reliable source to confirm that the dose is within the recommend range and then administer as ordered.

CHAPTER QUIZ

Convert weights and heights to the metric system and round to the nearest tenth. Round doses less than 1 mL to the nearest hundredth. Round doses greater than 1 mL to the nearest tenth. Round IV flow rates to the nearest whole number.

1. Convert 71 lb to kg.

   (A) 32.27 kg
   (C) 32.3 kg
   (B) 32.2 kg
   (D) 32.37 kg

2. Convert 5 feet 5 inches to cm.

   (A) 162.5 cm
   (C) 26 cm
   (B) 162.50 cm
   (D) 163.50 cm

3. Nipride 100 mg/250 mL D_5W. Calculate mcg/mL.

   (A) 200 mcg/mL
   (C) 0.4 mcg/mL
   (B) 400 mcg/mL
   (D) 2.5 mcg/mL

4. Patient: A 5-year-old child with Ewing's sarcoma; weight is 46 lb; height is 40 inches.

   Physician-ordered dose: Dactinomycin
   400 mcg/m²/day IV for 5 days
   What is the daily dose?

   (A) 232 mg   (C) 0.58 mcg

   (B) 0.76 m²   (D) 304 mcg

5. Patient: An 80-year-old man with hypertension; weight is 200 lb; height is 6 ft.

   Physician-ordered dose: Methyldopate
   2 g/m²/day

   (A) 4.3 g   (C) 4,360 mg

   (B) 4.26 g   (D) 4.3 mg

6. Patient: A 12-year old child; weight is 110 lb.

   Physician-ordered dose: Pentamidine 3 mg/kg daily

   Dose available: Pentamidine 60 mg/mL

   Using the formula method, calculate how much the nurse should administer for each dose.

   (A) 2.5 mL   (C) 2.25 mL

   (B) 2 mL   (D) 3 mL

7. Patient: A 50-year old woman; weight is 135 lb.

   Physician-ordered dose: Acyclovir 5 mg/kg every 8 hours for 7 days

   Dose available: Acyclovir 50 mg/mL

   Using the means:extremes method, calculate how much the nurse should administer for each dose.

   (A) 61.4 mL   (C) 6.2 mL

   (B) 6.14 mL   (D) 6.1 mL

8. Patient: A 58-year-old man; weight is 198 lb.

   Physician-ordered dose: Alpha-1 proteinase 60 mg/kg IV

   Dose available: Alpha-1 proteinase 20 mg/mL

   Using dimensional analysis, calculate how much the nurse should administer for each dose.

   (A) 27 mL   (C) 2.7 mL

   (B) 270 mL   (D) 0.27 mL

9. Physician-ordered dose: Nipride 4.5 mcg/kg/min

    Dose available: Nipride 50 mg/250 mL

    Patient weight = 65 kg

    Calculate the mL/hr.

    (A) 8.8 mL/hr   (C) 88 mL/hr

    (B) 87 mL/hr   (D) 87.75 mL/hr

10. Physician-ordered dose: Dobutamine hydrochloride
    4 mcg/kg/min

    Dose available: Dobutamine 250 mg/250 mL D$_5$W

    Patient weight = 150 lb

    Calculate the mL/hr.

    (A) 16 mL/hr   (C) 1.6 mL/hr

    (B) 160 mL/hr   (D) 16.3 mL/hr

ANSWERS AND EXPLANATIONS

1. C

Divide 71 lb by 2.2 to get kg: 71 ÷ 2.2 = 32.27.

Round to 32.3 kg.

2. A

Multiply the number of feet by 12 to get inches:
5 × 12 = 60.

Add 5 inches: 60 + 5 = 65 inches.

Multiply 65 inches by 2.5 to convert to cm:
65 × 2.5 = 162.5 cm.

3. B

Convert from mg/mL to mcg/mL by multiplying by 1,000.

$$\frac{\text{mg in solution} \times 1{,}000}{\text{total volume in mL}} \rightarrow \frac{100 \times 1{,}000}{250} = \frac{100{,}000 \text{ mcg}}{250 \text{ mL}}$$

Reduce this fraction to lowest terms: 100,000 mcg ÷ 250 mL = 400 mcg/mL. There are 400 mcg per mL.

4. D

STEP 1: Convert patient weight to kg and round to the tenth: 46 ÷ 2.2 = 20.909090 → 20.9 kg.

STEP 2: Convert patient height to cm and round to the tenth: 40 × 2.5 = 100 cm (no rounding needed).

STEP 3: Calculate patient body surface area using the formula.

$$\text{BSA} = \sqrt{\frac{\text{height in cm} \times \text{weight in kg}}{3{,}600 \text{ (constant) m}^2 \text{ (square meters)}}}$$

$$\text{BSA} = \sqrt{\frac{100 \text{ cm} \times 20.9 \text{ kg}}{3{,}600 \text{ m}^2}} = 0.76 \text{ m}^2$$

The patient's body surface area is 0.76 m².

STEP 4: Calculate the desired dose.

Multiply the BSA of 0.76 m² by 400 to determine the ordered dose: 0.76 × 400 = 304 mcg (no rounding needed).

The total ordered dose is 304 mcg.

5.   A

STEP 1: Convert patient weight to kg and round to the tenth: $200 \div 2.2 = 90.909090 \rightarrow 90.9$ kg.

STEP 2: Convert patient height to cm and round to the tenth. Convert 6 feet to inches: $6 \times 12 = 72$ inches.

Convert inches to cm: $72 \times 2.5 = 180$ cm (no rounding needed).

STEP 3: Calculate patient BSA.

$$BSA = \sqrt{\frac{180 \text{ cm} \times 90.9 \text{ kg}}{3{,}600 \text{ m}^2}} = 2.13 \text{ m}^2$$

The patient's body surface area is 2.13 m².

STEP 4: Calculate the desired dose.

Multiply the BSA of 2.13 m² by 2 g and round to determine the ordered dose: $2.13 \times 2 = 4.26 \rightarrow 4.3$ g. The total ordered dose is 4.3 g.

6.   A

Convert 110 lb to kg: $100 \div 2.2 = 50$ kg.

Multiply 50 by 3 mg/kg to determine the ordered dose: $50 \times 3 = 150$.

The total ordered dose is 150 mg.

Formula method

$$\text{desired} \rightarrow \frac{150 \text{ mg}}{60 \text{ mg}} \times 1 \text{ mL} \leftarrow \text{quantity}$$
$$\text{have} \rightarrow$$

Divide: $150 \div 60 = 2.5$

Multiply: $2.5 \times 1 \text{ mL} = 2.5$ mL

The nurse should administer 2.5 mL to the patient.

7.   D

Convert 135 lb to kg and round: $135 \div 2.2 = 61.363 \rightarrow 61.4$ kg.

Multiply 61.4 by 5 mg/kg to determine the ordered dose: $61.4 \times 5 = 307$.

The total ordered dose is 307 mg.

(mg/mL available) 50 mg : 1 mL = 307 mg : x mL (ordered dose/unknown mL)

(multiply the means) $307 = 50x$ (multiply the extremes)

(divide both sides by 50) $307 \div 50 = 50x \div 50$

$6.14 = x$

Round to 6.1 mL. The nurse should administer 6.1 mL to the patient.

8. B

Convert 198 lb to kg: 198 ÷ 2.2 = 90 kg.

Multiply 90 by 60 mg to determine the ordered dose: 90 × 60 = 5,400.

The ordered dose is 5,400 mg.

$$x = \frac{5,400 \text{ mg}}{1} \times \frac{1 \text{ mL}}{20 \text{ mg}}$$

Cancel out the duplicate labels and multiply straight across.

$$x = \frac{5,400}{1} \times \frac{1 \text{ mL}}{20} = \frac{5,400 \text{ ml}}{20} \quad \begin{array}{l} \text{(multiply the numerators)} \\ \text{(multiply the denominators)} \end{array}$$

Divide the products: 5,400 ÷ 20 = 270.

The nurse should administer 270 mL to the patient.

9. C

The weight is stated in kilograms.

Convert the available dose from mg/mL to mcg/mL (multiply by 1,000) and reduce to lowest terms.

$$\begin{array}{l} \text{mg in solution} \times 1,000 \rightarrow \\ \text{total volume in mL} \rightarrow \end{array} \frac{50 \times 1,000}{250} = \frac{50,000 \text{ mcg}}{250 \text{ mL}} = \frac{200 \text{ mcg}}{1 \text{ mL}}$$

There are 200 mcg/mL.

Set up the equation to determine mL/hr to equal mcg/kg/min.

$$\frac{4.5 \text{ mcg/kg/min} \times 60 \text{ min/hr} \times 65 \text{ kg}}{200 \text{ mcg/mL}}$$

Cross off the labels, multiply, and reduce to lowest terms.

$$\frac{4.5 \times 60 \times 65}{200} = \frac{17,550}{200} = 87.75$$

Round to the nearest whole number. The nurse should set the electronic infusion device at 88 mL/hr to deliver 4.5 mcg/kg/min.

10. A

Convert the patient's weight from pounds to kilograms and round to the tenth: $150 \div 2.2 = 68.18 \rightarrow 68.2$ kg.

Convert the available dose from mg/mL to mcg/mL (multiply by 1,000) and reduce to lowest terms.

$$\frac{\text{mg in solution} \times 1,000 \rightarrow}{\text{total volume in mL} \rightarrow} \quad \frac{250 \times 1,000}{250} = \frac{250,000 \text{ mcg}}{250 \text{ mL}} = \frac{1,000 \text{ mcg}}{1 \text{ mL}}$$

There are 1,000 mcg/mL.

Set up the equation to determine mL/hr to equal mcg/kg/min.

$$\frac{4 \text{ mcg/kg/min} \times 60 \text{ min/hr} \times 68.2 \text{ kg}}{1,000 \text{ mcg/mL}}$$

Cross off the labels, multiply, and reduce to lowest terms.

$$\frac{4 \times 60 \times 68.2}{1,000} = \frac{16,368}{1,000} = 16.368$$

Round to the nearest whole number. The nurse should set the electronic infusion device at 16 mL/hr to deliver 4 mcg/kg/min.